THE
MAKEOVER
BOOK

Also by the Author:
Celebrity Style Secrets

Jacqui Ripley is a freelance journalist who writes for *Hello!*, *InStyle*, *Cosmopolitan*, *Zest*, the *Standard*, the *Sunday Express* and *New Woman*. She lives in East London.

THE
MAKEOVER
BOOK

Simple Ideas for Effortless Style

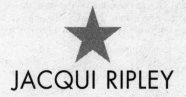

JACQUI RIPLEY

PIATKUS

For my mother Hazel

✿ *Visit the Piatkus website!*

Piatkus publishes a wide range of best-selling fiction and non-fiction, including books on health, mind, body & spirit, sex, self-help, cookery, biography and the paranormal.

If you want to:

- read descriptions of our popular titles
- buy our books over the Internet
- take advantage of our special offers
- enter our monthly competition
- learn more about your favourite Piatkus authors

VISIT OUR WEBSITE AT: www.piatkus.co.uk

Copyright © 2004 by Jacqui Ripley
First published in 2004 by
Piatkus Books Ltd
5 Windmill Street
London W1T 2JA

e-mail: info@piatkus.co.uk

The moral right of the author has been asserted

A catalogue record for this book is available from the British Library

ISBN 0 7499 2571 X

Text design by Goldust Design
Edited by Lizzie Hutchins

This book has been printed on paper manufactured with respect for the environment using wood from managed sustainable resources

Set by Action Publishing Technology Ltd, Gloucester
Printed and bound in Denmark by
Nørhaven Paperback A/S, Viborg

Contents

Acknowledgements

I was originally inspired to write this book not by the rash of television programmes ordering you to look better but by reading *Sleeping Beauties* by the wonderful, insightful and always irreverent Mavis Cheek. The book revolves around the comings and goings of Tabitha's Beauty Parlour, where clients are given the makeovers of their lives, with very unexpected and often very funny results. Setting the delights of good writing and humour to one side, I decided to write this book because I really do believe that a makeover, however big or small, can be a catalyst for change to the point where you never look back and only move forwards.

Thanks go to my agent, Teresa Chris, for her genuine enthusiasm, Alice Davis, my editor at Piatkus, for making the whole process seem so simple, my husband John (as always) and my son Dylan.

Introduction

'There are no ugly women, only lazy ones.'
Helena Rubinstein

I adore this quote. You know why? Because I think it's true. Every single woman possesses an inner fabulousness, whether she's aware of it or not. And this is what this book is all about – encouraging you to rethink your top-to-toe style and ultimately reward yourself with a new and infinitely improved you. It's about taking a little time out from your day to give yourself the Star Treatment. Believe me, a complete makeover – and I'm not talking new noses, brow lifts, cheeks and breast implants, but easy, 100 per cent do-able tips, tricks and beauty buys – will deliver more effortless style, beauty and health into your life.

Makeover – just the word is enough to give divine inspiration. Everybody loves a great makeover, whether it involves dropping a few pounds or knocking five years off your age with a new hair colour. And I guarantee you'll never tire of people telling you how great you look.

If this sounds like a whole lot of work, then be reassured it isn't. My makeover philosophy is simple: stand back and have an outer body experience with yourself. By this I mean look at yourself objectively in every tiny detail, from the stray hairs that need plucking under your brows to the habitual slobbing around in old clothes at the weekend, and ask yourself: 'Am I making the most of myself?' If the answer is a resounding 'No', then it's time to remake yourself to order.

This book is not about rules, it's about making small changes and getting big results. It's problem solving at its very best – chucking out the old and bringing in the new (you). It's about becoming your own stylist, facialist, nutritionist, hairdresser and personal trainer all rolled into one.

Your appearance says a lot about you and how you value yourself. We don't like to admit that we judge people on the way they look, but we do. So, what does your image really say about you? How do you feel about it? Remember how you feel when you come out of the hairdresser's? Or when you're wearing something special? You feel amazing, more confident, keen to be noticed. Just think how it would be to have that feeling every day rather than just on the few occasions when you take the time to think about yourself. It all comes down to taking control. Take over yourself and you begin to makeover yourself.

Lots of women are intimidated by the idea of style. They think it's a mystical art. But I can assure you it's not. In my role as a beauty and fashion journalist I've learned from the experts that the difference between ordinary and extra-ordinary can literally be down to such simple things as skirt length or the way you wear your hair.

In this book I aim to demystify style and reveal the real secret of looking and feeling great. So start turning these pages and read on. Soon you'll be hair happy forever, loving good-for-you-food and just dying to open your wardrobe and put on all your lovely clothes. Before you know it, your makeover will be giving you the confidence to shout: 'Where are the parties?'

quiz

DO YOU NEED A MAKEOVER?
Do you really need a makeover? How would you know if you did? Take this quiz to find out.

1. You haven't changed your hair colour since:
a) High school. And you're proud of it.
b) Over a year ago. Or was it two?
c) Three months ago. Your colourist is on speed dial.

2. Your Little Black Dress is:
a) For life.
b) For funerals.
c) A garment to be bought each season.

3. Who is your style inspiration?
a) Your grandmother. Pearls are such a good look.
b) Your mother. You admire her recycling skills.
c) Movie greats such as Lauren Bacall.

4. Your essential take-everywhere make-up bag contains:
a) The absolute basics: mascara, concealer and lipgloss.
b) Two lipsticks (daytime sheer and vampy for evening) and a powder compact.

c) Three eyeshadow quartets, four lipsticks, concealer, mascara and eyelash curler.

5. Which workout are you currently doing?

a) Jane 'Feel the burn' Fonda.

b) Pilates.

c) Bikram Yoga.

6. You arrive for a dinner date with a new man. He says:

a) 'Did you come straight from the office/school run/local church meeting?'

b) 'I'm always attracted to women who remind me of my mother.'

c) 'Yeah, baby! Bring it on!'

7. When you walk into a party:

a) People ask you for a drink.

b) You get your own drink.

c) Men offer to shake you a cocktail.

8. You dress to:

a) Keep warm.

b) Blend into the background.

c) Thrill.

9. Your favourite look is:

a) Spray-on stonewashed jeans tucked into tight boots.

b) A crisp white shirt and a sleek black skirt.

c) No fuss or flounce but a scene-stealing statement-making jacket or skirt.

10. Your style motto is:

a) If it ain't broke, don't fix it.

b) Always make-up and never make-do.

c) Change is for the better.

YOUR SCORE:
Mostly As

When was the last time you let your lips loose on a colour stronger than your own? I'm stunned you've reached womanhood without the first clue on how to work your feminine, let alone your wild side. Your number one priority should be not making over your garden or your living room, but yourself. As a make-up virgin, start slowly on building up your new look, as you won't feel entirely comfortable going from nude to knockout in minutes. Focus on either the eyes or lips and take it from there.

Mostly Bs

If *you're* bored with your well-worn look, how can you expect others to be excited? Whatever fashion revival is going on now, you can be sure you're still wearing it from first time round. Take action: life, not to mention style, evolves, and that means wearing a different hairstyle from the one you flicked at your graduation. Chuck out that pink frosty lipstick that reminds you of your very first kiss and update your make-up with new colours and textures. You'll be surprised how it will move on your look and throw you head first into the 21st century.

Mostly Cs

Wow! Your look is hot, hotter, hottest. The only reason you must have picked up this book is to pass it on to a friend who's a serious embarrassment to walk out the door with. You eagerly digest the current make-up trends and what you don't know about style isn't worth knowing. You love experimenting and your ideal Saturday would be spent gliding around a fashion-led department store, while your idea of a disaster would be being caught without your lash-building mascara. But a word of warning: don't fall into the trap of becoming a fashion victim. Perhaps the word 'makeunder' should come into play now and again.

WARNING

**YOU ARE ABOUT TO
ENTER A MAKE-UP ZONE.**

**PLEASE ADJUST
YOUR LOOK.**

WARNING

YOU ARE ABOUT TO
ENTER A MAKEUP ZONE

PLEASE ADJUST
YOUR LOOK.

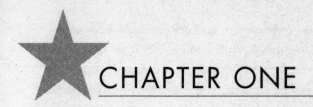

CHAPTER ONE

Making way for great skin

'Nature gives you the face you have at 20. It's up to you to merit the face you have at 50.'
Coco Chanel

There are plenty of things you can't change in your life, but the condition of your skin isn't one of them. And I'm not talking paralysing frown lines with Botox or plumping out wrinkles with fillers, I'm talking a simple but clever skincare plan that will give fabulous results.

Yes, you can have a great-looking skin without spending megabucks or precious hours performing an addictive 12-step skincare regime. The skin gurus I've met and interviewed over the years all agree: treat your complexion with respect and in return it will reward you with a locked-in luminous glow. Cosmetic surgery aside, many facialists truly believe that by becoming a devotee of your own skin – that's knowing how to evaluate and treat it – you will notice a big improvement in just three months.

And don't believe that a radiant complexion is all in the genes. Of course, there's a certain amount of God-given luck dished out in the complexion department, but that's certainly not the whole story. I've learned that giving time to your skin is the key. It doesn't have to be a ritual that's complicated, just consistent. A professional facial can be priceless in the short term, but it's the home care in between that counts.

How is your skincare routine right now? Does it need a makeover? Just as we can cling onto a certain hairstyle, so our skincare can get stuck in a time warp too. Are you still religiously hanging onto the type of moisturiser you had five or ten years ago? With skincare now becoming ever more sophisticated, there's really no excuse not to rethink your routine. And if your skin is young enough to be effortlessly luminous, it's about acting now and not paying the beauty penalty later.

Put simply, ageing isn't an affliction that hits between 25 and 45, it's the accumulated effects of the way you have treated or mistreated your skin over the course of your life. Genetics notwithstanding, maintaining great skin takes a little bit of work at every age. So figure out the best way to start right here, with a dose of the latest in skin wisdom.

How to buy great-looking skin

What busy woman doesn't want perfect skin all tied up in one supermarket shop? But cruising the skincare aisles these days is like drooling over the display in a patisserie. Everything looks so tempting. How do you choose between a chocolate éclair and a strawberry cream-filled tart? Or between a cleanser and a moisturiser? How do you figure out what you actually need?

A real problem

A friend recently said to me: 'I walked into a department store with the aim of buying a super-duper cream to give me cashmere-feeling skin. I was faced with a cluster of efficient-looking women standing behind all these skin counters, looking like they had beamed down from the planet Vulcan. I felt completely intimidated and walked straight out. Does it really have to be this much of a struggle to get a better-looking complexion?'

Well, yes and no. The struggle is personal. Over

time and through trial and error, we cobble together a hotch-potch of lotions that we think work. Along the way we may have bought a few other products on the advice of a friend or invested in a cream that promised to send wrinkles into submission. In short, it can all be very random and chaotic. But the makeover lesson here is that if you're logical and goal-oriented it doesn't have to be.

EVALUATE YOUR SKIN TYPE

First things first: cosmetic research now emphasises that skin no longer falls under the rigid and traditional categories of normal, oily and dry. Although these still stand, they are to be viewed as very broad categories and within them are common and very modern problems such as fine lines, irritation, sensitivity, dullness and general pore misbehaviour. The skin makeover rule here is to think of your skin as ever-changing.

Climate, sun, diet, physical damage, heartbreak, stress and ageing all cause changes to your skin. Where you live, work and relax also has a significant impact. There's 'city skin', for instance, characteristically with a congested appearance, maybe a sallow tinge, a tendency towards breakouts caused by pollution and air conditioning, and a lack of vibrancy from the negative ions released by computer screens. Then there's 'workout skin', where the gym may be great for your body but not so pleasing for the skin. Flaky, itchy patches may arise from chlorine in the swimming pool or too much sweating may result in a tight, uncomfortable feeling to the skin. And then there's 'the-great-outdoors skin', which is a dry complexion and a tendency towards high colour and broken capillaries on the cheeks from spending a lot of time outside.

★ **TIME TO DITCH** *Aggressive skincare in winter if your complexion is fragile. The skin is drier and more sensitive then because of indoor heating and low humidity.*

★ **CHANGE IT NOW** *Leave harsher treatments (peels) until the spring.*

ARE YOU READY TO GLOW?

Know your skin type and a basic skincare formula will naturally follow. But it cannot be stressed enough that you should adjust your skincare routine regularly and not assume that your skin's needs remain constant. Get-you-gorgeous skin all boils down to two words: *being adapt-able*.

If you frequently monitor your skin, it will stand a great chance of looking good no matter what its issues are. What might these issues be?

Dehydrated Skin

Description: Any skin type can fall prey to dehydration. Don't be fooled that oily skin can't suffer from a bout of thirst – it can. Dehydrated skin is caused by exposure to weather extremes (hot or cold), illness and stress. It looks dull and feels taut or slightly itchy. A test is to put your fingers across the bottom of your cheek and gently press upwards. Any fine horizontal lines indicate a dehydrated skin.

Make it over: Moisture creams give skin immediate relief. Hardworking ingredients, specifically humectants (moisture trappers), grab humidity from the air and hold the water in the skin. Hydrating masks are a quick fix and serums can be slotted into your daycare during this high and dry time for an added moisture surge.

Dry Skin

Description: Dry skin looks tight, dull and flaky due to a lack of sebum. It dries out fast in the sun, wind and cold and can look aged before its time if not respected. Dry skin can be confused with dehydrated skin, but whereas parched skin feels instantly better with a slathering of moisture, dry skin will feel as though it needs more.

Make it over: Opt for an extra-creamy cleanser and avoid toners containing alcohol, as they can have a real drying effect on skin. For a moisturiser, look for concentrated formulas. In the long term these can make a real difference to dryness. Exfoliate regularly: dead skin cells (which look like dry flaky skin) can prevent moisture from reaching the subcutaneous (deeper) layers of the skin. Drink plenty of water.

Normal Skin

Description: The skin we would all love to have. Normal skin efficiently regulates its own pH balance, which blesses it with a texture that's neither too oily nor too dry, and it has few blemishes.

Make it over: All you need is to keep it simple. Cleanse with a water-based cleanser and moisturise lightly, except in extreme conditions. Regular exfoliation will keep cell renewal on target too.

Stressed Skin

Description: A stressed skin is one suffering from flaking, blotching and blemishes. Any skin type can be stressed due to a whole combination of things, including anxiety, pollution and harsh weather.

Make it over: Use protective products to soothe the skin. Look for buzzwords such as 'comforting' and 'relaxing'. A night cream can give over-the-edge skin plenty of TLC too.

Oily Skin

Description: Shininess, open pores and blackheads sum up an oily skin. This skin produces too much sebum (oil) and can be brought on by humidity or hormonal fluctuations. In the long term, though, it ages more slowly, so it's not all bad news.

Make it over: The wrong choice of product can make a huge difference and with oily skin tending to attract more dirt than dry, it's crucial to get the cleansing balance right. Anything that contains alcohol will strip the skin and result in an overproduction of sebum, making oily skin worse. This skin craves a gentle touch, so look for specific products to redress the oil balance. Opt for non-comedogenic (non pore-blocking) formulas. If you are prone to breakouts, look for products containing benzoyl peroxide and just dab them onto spots – not slather on the whole face.

Combination Skin

Description: This skin has a split personality. One part may be dry while another is oily. The term 'T-zone' refers to combination skin where the forehead, nose and chin are oily but the cheeks and the area around the eyes are dry.

Make it over: The trick with this kind of condition is to find products that will keep your skin hydrated while minimising breakouts and shine in the oily areas. Look for a light cleanser designed for combination skin and graduate the use of moisturiser according to the area of the face. Products that boast alpha hydroxy acids and vitamin A retinols can also help balance this type of skin.

Sensitive Skin

Description: Many dermatologists believe that sensitive skin is made, not born, and is much on the increase due to the lifestyle we lead. Illness, stress or chemical insult can all set off a sensitive reaction, which can range from itching and swelling to soreness and roughness.

Make it over: Before buying creams, scan the ingredients. The fewer, the better. The most common irritants include fragrance, isopropyl alcohol, dyes, PABA, lanolin, sorbic acid, formaldehyde and benzoic acid. Test samples on your neck for a few days and see how your skin reacts. And keep products to a minimum: each will harbour around 20 to 40 ingredients, so even just using four a day will subject your complexion to several hundred different chemical substances. Look for the buzzword 'hypoallergenic'.

Ageing Skin

Description: It's said that there are three major factors involved in skin ageing: chronological, environmental and hormonal ageing. All of these give rise to a skin that has a noticeable loss of firmness and looks and acts fatigued. And to add insult to injury, in the ten years following the menopause, collagen levels fall by 30 per cent as a result of oestrogen deficiency and skin dryness becomes an increasing problem.

Make it over: Here you need a two-prong approach. First, preventative skincare is key. It's estimated that up to 80 per cent of premature ageing is caused by UV light, so moisturisers with an added SPF, preferably 15, should be used. Secondly, the over thirties should consider adding at least one 'active' product to their daily routine. 'Active' means with ingredients in a strong enough concentration to produce visible changes in texture and quality. Vitamins A, C and AHAs (alpha hydroxy acids) are widely considered to be the mainstays of an efficient anti-ageing regime.

ESSENTIAL STEPS TO SKIN SHOPPING SUCCESS

Women with beautiful complexions usually have very definite and clear-cut opinions about skincare. And like people who believe they've found the only path to enlightenment, they tend to be extremists. So, whether it's putting their radiant and plumped up epidermis down to never going in the sun, rubbing yoghurt on their faces or drinking their own urine (yes really!), they all have a definite skincare programme.

Now, I'm not saying yours has to be as intense, but assemble key products that work for your needs (being guided by the skin descriptions above), use them flexibly and you'll be well on your way to having your own gorgeous skin. But the secret is not to become a product junkie and be seduced into changing your routine every five minutes, as that can leave skin feeling confused. Clinical trials show that products are more effective when used consistently for three months or longer.

When introducing new products, do so one at a time and allow your skin two weeks to adjust. To help you through, here's a counter intelligence guide to the basic products you need to keep your skin functioning well and looking its best.

Cleanser

To keep skin looking healthy, it's necessary to rid it of the grime, make-up and other particles that will cover it after a day's exposure to the environment. If you don't, it will render all additional skincare less effective. But the importance of this first get-great-skin step is often overlooked, which, believe me, is many a skin's downfall. Some experts go as far to say that if cleansing is done incorrectly, it's one of the most damaging things you can do to your skin. So how should you go about it?

As a general guideline: use a gentle milky formula if you have dry or sensitive skin and a foam or oil-free gel if you have oily skin. Ultimately skin should feel comfortable after cleaning, never tight or burning. Please your skin's senses and that way you won't skip this vital task.

Toner

A toner's job is to remove cleanser residue, regulate the pH balance of the skin and leave it feeling mountain-stream fresh.

Whether to tone or not to tone has always been a debate amongst skincare specialists. Many oily skins find toners beneficial, as they calm oil glands, but normal, dry and sensitive skins can afford to skip them and use pure rose-water (from any chemist) as an alternative to a more expensive toner.

Moisturiser

At its most basic moisturiser helps keep the skin soft and supple by providing a physical barrier that insulates it from the elements. As the first signs of ageing hit – a lacklustre skin and fine wrinkles – look for formulas stuffed with antioxidants (vitamins A, C and E along with green tea).

A major un-dewing of the skin is the sun – although it gives life, it also leeches water out of the skin. For any skin type, wearing a daytime moisturiser with SPF 15 is recommended. Even oily skin needs moisture, if only on those areas that are dry.

Serums give dry, tired or stressed skins a concentrated moisture boost that produces both an immediate result (glowing skin) and a cumulative action (a more resilient complexion). Creams marketed as being 'Botox like' may provide visible results, as they have the formulas to soften and slow down muscle contraction.

Night Cream

It's tempting to think that we need both a day *and* night cream only to make skin companies richer, however there are proven differences in skin activity from day to night. During the day, skin faces a multitude of challenges that affect cellular activity. At night, it is freed of external damage and the cells devote their time to recovering their basic functions. So skin metabolism is working while you're in the land of nod and is more receptive to treatments you apply before hitting the pillow.

Skin boffins recommend using both a day and night cream as they work synergistically to keep skin functioning at its optimum. Look for ones with potent antioxidants such as white tea and soy.

Skin Brighteners

Sometimes classed as 'hero' products, these illuminators work by evening out the skin tone. Applied under make-up, they rebalance, retexture and reinvigorate the complexion by fading areas of discoloration. They are perfect for skins with sun damage or pigmentation problems, or for bringing much-needed radiance to a skin that's partied a little too hard.

Skin Firmers

Dermatologists agree these can be great quick fixes before hitting the town. Firming products trap water in your skin. Technically they don't really firm the skin – creams can only go so far! – but they do make it appear more plumped up and address the loss of elasticity that leads to skin slackening over time. In essence, they deliver water and seal it in promptly, thereby swelling up cells and making fine lines less noticeable – momentarily. The skin will appear more taut, but alas it's only a Cinderella scenario – the effect usually lasts no more than a few hours.

Masks

Most face masks work on the premise that they're a top-up for your skin when it craves a little extra help. Think of them as yoga for the skin – they visibly relax and nourish the skin and in just 10 minutes you can see the difference.

Keep a 'wardrobe' of masks to hand, depending on how your skin's reacting: a deep cleansing clay mask when a regular cleanse just isn't enough to draw impurities out from a 'city' skin; a hydrating mask when skin is feeling high and dry; and a rescue or relaxing mask for when skin is out of sorts.

For optimum results, cleanse the face and apply mask pre-bath, then soak and remove post-bathing. Steam will help the active ingredients to penetrate the skin.

Face Peels

Exfoliation makes your skin appear plump and juicy. Why? Because polishing up the skin eliminates dead cells from the surface and therefore improves skin smoothness and luminosity. Skin that is well buffed will drink up moisture so much better. There's no great science behind it: you are simply helping your skin to do what it does naturally.

Now, going beyond a simple physical exfoliation scrub, skincare companies have got clever, taken inspiration from procedures used by cosmetic dermatologists in their clinics and whipped up multi-factorial well-researched ways of making your skin look more radiant with at-home peels. These can either contain highly refined aluminium oxide crystals to gently remove the top layer of the skin (referred to as microdermabrasion), chemical exfoliants that boast acid formulas such as salicylic acid that work by dissolving the protein bond that keeps old cells attached to the skin, or biological formulas that contain ingredients of tropical fruit enzymes – think papaya, mango and pineapple – to lift loose skin cells clean away. However, be warned: although these do-it-yourself treatments can be effective, skin doctors recommend reading the directions carefully. Those with skin upsets such as redness, inflamed blemishes such as cystic acne and eczema should avoid face peels. As a guideline: if your skin cannot tolerate normal exfoliators, do not use stronger formulas.

Eye Creams

Research reveals that two thirds of all women worry about crow's feet and half worry about dark circles under their eyes. The skin around the eyes is a quarter of the thickness of skin on the rest of the face and is consequently more delicate. Eyes are focused on much incidental abuse too: the removal of mascara, smoke-filled rooms, popping contact lenses and crying! And don't think you can cheat and get away with patting an extra bit of your face lotion underneath your eyes. You can't. These formulas are too thick and too rich and can lead to puffiness as well as small whiteheads (milia) beneath the skin. Eye creams are formulated to be milder and less irritating for this delicate area. Just apply them with care. Use the tip of your small finger and gently massage in a clockwise circle around the lid and underneath the eye.

How your skin faces up to ageing

Personally I have to agree with Lauren Hutton, a former Revlon face, who states, 'The point of life should be to grow up. If we start hiding because we turned 40 or 45, well, we should get a good spanking.'

But that said, ageing can be hard to face. A study conducted among women aged 30 to 45 revealed that until the age of 30 women generally apply a simple facial moisturiser, principally to avoid the skin feeling tight. But when, from the age of 30, the skin begins to undergo noticeable changes, women rarely feel ready to move on to an anti-wrinkle cream. This is essentially for psychological reasons: they prove reticent to start using an anti-ageing product. They have the feeling of passing a point of no return. Is that you?

Choosing the correct treatment for your age can be confusing. But the decision can be crucial. Here is a dermatological insight into how the skin ages as it passes through each decade. With this information you can decide how best to update your regime to put your best face forwards.

TIME TO DITCH *The Peter Pan skin factor.*

 CHANGE IT NOW *Upgrade your skincare according to your age.*

TWENTIES
Skin mantra: Prime time

High levels of hormones mean that your skin is at its most resilient and elastic now. Wrinkles are virtually non-existent.

Skin prescription:
★ Look for cleansers that control oil.
★ Pick up a moisturiser with a sun protection factor (SPF). Sun damage incurred now will show up in ten years' time.

THIRTIES
Skin mantra: Keeping up appearances

Eye crinkles, broken capillaries and sun spots can all be evident now. The skin begins to look less like a well-sprung mattress and feels drier.

Skin prescription:
★ Target your efforts into using an effective moisturiser with a potent source of antioxidants to protect your skin from free radicals as well as keeping the top skin layers smooth and hydrated.
★ A night cream with retinol will help boost your collagen reserves.
★ If skin is looking dull, introduce it to a brightener or a more efficient exfoliating campaign.
★ Start using an eye cream.

FORTIES

Skin mantra: The mid-life slow down

Hormone changes associated with the menopause mean skin is less firm and resilient now and may be subject to flare-ups you thought were over in your teens.

Skin prescription:

★ If you haven't been using a retinol treatment (vitamin A) do so now, as it will stimulate the cells and increase collagen production.

★ The skin is now lazier, so exfoliation or face peels are key for a brighter-looking complexion.

FIFTIES AND BEYOND

Skin mantra: Protect and survive

Declining levels of oestrogen affect the skin's elasticity, pigment, firmness and tone. The skin loses up to 30 per cent of collagen in the first five years of the menopause.

Skin prescription:

★ Intensive moisturisers that encourage cell renewal and help restore elasticity should be an integral part of your routine.

★ Look for super-firming complexes and serums and, most importantly, creams rich in isoflavones or phytoestrogens. These are plant molecules that resemble human hormones and can work in their place to stimulate collagen and elastic activity in the skin. Just think of them as cell energisers.

How to be your own dermatologist

The first and most important step in any skincare treatment is the analysis of your skin. When you see a dermatologist or even a facialist, they will use more than their naked eye to assess your skin. They will scrutinise it section by section, using both a magnifying lamp and touch. This will then throw up clues as to how and why your skin is behaving as it is.

According to the art of Chinese face reading, your health is written all over your face. In the same way that areas of the feet are related to health in the practice of reflexology, so areas or zones of the face are related to internal organs. The idea is to use the face as a map.

For a Chinese takeaway diagnostic face reading, check out these areas:

The kidneys: The half-moon shaped area under the eye Working too hard and eating too many rich foods will cause an imbalance in the fluid balance of the body. If you're hungover with worry or have been drinking too much coffee, this area will be puffy and blue. Look at your ears too: if they are redder than the skin on your face, you are overworking your adrenal glands.

The liver: The middle of the forehead between the eyebrows
If this area is dark brown and has a congested look your liver is throwing up signs of 'liver energy stagnation'. This could mean that it is stressed. Causes could include frustration, rich food and alcohol. Spots and lines on the forehead indicate congestion from too much oily food or dairy. Eat more wholefoods and up your water intake.

The stomach and intestines: The mouth and the lower part of the face
The mouth highlights the energy of the stomach and intestines and the lower part of the face relates to the lower abdomen. Congestion such as white spots or a granular-like feel under the skin, along with blotchy areas, may indicate a yeast infection from too much dairy or sugar in the diet. If the chin is red and swollen, it may mean there is a structural weakness in the organs or candida. If the top lip is cracked, red or has spots at the corners, this could point to stomach acidity or heat caused by inappropriate diet.

The lungs: The cheeks
Redness, puffiness and breakouts on one or both cheeks indicate too many dairy products that produce mucus and congestion in the lungs or respiratory distress from smoking. You may be on the verge of a bronchial infection if this area suddenly becomes red and dry.

DEAR SKIN DIARY

Like our hearts, our skin can become emotional. More dermatologists and skin specialists are recognising that it is an organ of emotional expression and often it's trying to express some unresolved internal tension. Test the theory and keep a Bridget Jones-style skin diary.

- ★ *Monday:* Overstretched at work = oily complexion.
- ★ *Tuesday:* Called in by boss and given a rollicking = blotchy skin.
- ★ *Wednesday:* Very important social event = spots on nose.
- ★ *Thursday:* A family fallout = flaring up of old eczema problem.
- ★ *Friday:* Win the lottery, resign from job and make up with family = blissfully happy skin.

This, of course, is fiction! But you can see how being on a rollercoaster of emotions can trouble your skin. Chemical changes bought on by tension and anxiety may provoke breakouts or acne and has commonly been referred to as 'super-achiever skin'. And it's ever more frequent in 30-something women.

How to Uncover your Emotional Triggers

It's easier to deal with a skin problem when you know what's going on emotionally. If you treat dry skin or spots without acknowledging the underlying cause, you're missing the point.

So, does your skin need a shrink? If you suspect that there may be an emotional link to your skin condition, keep a (sensible) skin diary where you record your daily ups and downs, activities and skin status. Jot down good, bad and seemingly non-eventful events. At the end of a month you may notice a pattern to your stress and skin upsets. Don't be surprised if there's a lapse of several days between the emotional event and your skin flare-up. Record-keeping may give you some insight into what kind of upset, pressure or stress triggers your skin problem.

A bad case of continually miserable skin may well need professional help beyond the skin counter – you may even benefit from therapy from a psychologist. Learning to understand the emotions that affect your skin can help you take control of a situation that is mirrored in your skin. And through time, various relaxation techniques or self-acceptance, the condition can clear up – for good.

A real problem

Researchers have also looked at the stress-induced release of a specific substance in the body as a triggering factor for psoriasis. As a case in point an old work colleague of mine had a terrible flare-up of psoriasis the day before she got married. Her GP prescribed her a cream to calm her harassed skin down, she dutifully went up the aisle and was separated less than 18 months later. Perhaps she should have 'read' her skin and realised that maybe he wasn't her true love match!

ARE YOU GUILTY OF SKIN CRIMES?

On a good day our skin can make us feel like facing the world without a trace of translucent powder and on a bad day – well, let's just call it a duvet day. But sometimes we only have ourselves to blame for skin that's less radiant than a 100 watt lightbulb. If you thought squeezing the odd spot was the only skin crime you could commit, well, think again. Assault and battery are regular crimes committed on innocent pores every day.

What's the use of making over your skincare routine if you've still not kicked the habits that are cramping your complexion's style? Scan your eyes down the six skin offences that are positively criminal and if you are guilty as charged, read on for smart ways of getting parole.

1. Picking and Squeezing Spots

Hands up who hasn't squeezed spots and I will class you as a saint. Once there, spots are hard to ignore. But according to the British Dermatological Association, squeezing them, especially at an early stage, will just push the inflammation further into the skin, resulting in a bigger spot. Picking the tops off spots will also introduce other infections from your nail as well as scarring.

Parole points: Dab the offending spot(s) with a salicylic acid gel or cream – available in formulations over the counter – twice a day. This will help dry out the spot in under a week.

If a whitehead forms, you can extract the pus to limit the damage, but only in the right way. Take a piece of cotton wool, soak it in warm water, then hold it over the whitehead for a few seconds. Then wrap your two index fingers in tissues and press down gently around the blemish for a few seconds until it disperses. Disinfect the area either with a dab of tea tree oil or an antibacterial solution.

2. A Diet High in Sugar

The skin is made up of structural proteins such as elastin and collagen fibres and dermatologists know that sugar can attach itself chemically to a whole variety of elements, including protein. So the more sugar you have in your body, the more likely it is that sugar will be attaching itself to protein. This is very harmful to the skin. Here's why: if the elastic fibres of the skin are bound to sugar, they won't be as flexible and may be more prone to deterioration. For instance, if an enzyme that repairs skin after sun exposure isn't working properly because it's got sugar stuck to it, then that important function isn't going to happen.

Parole points: Keep in mind that the body converts anything that's starch into sugar, so cut out as many refined carbohydrates as possible. These are classed as high glycaemic index foods. Sticking to low glycaemic index foods (meat, fish and pulses) will give you energy that is released slowly, so you will be less reliant on foods that give a quick sugar rush.

3. Smoking

Every cigarette contains 4,000 toxins, many of which are carried by the bloodstream into the dermis (deeper layer) of the skin. In fact smoking exerts such a noticeable effect on the skin that it's possible to detect whether or not a person is a smoker just by looking at them. Smokers have more wrinkles around the eyes and mouth and their skin tends to have a greyish pallor.

Now scientists think they may have discovered why smokers look older than non-smokers. A study by dermatologists published in *The Lancet* a couple of years ago showed that smoking activates the genes responsible for an enzyme that breaks down collagen in the skin. When this starts to disintegrate, skin begins to sag and wrinkle.

Parole points: If you smoke, you're likely to be wasting your money on anti-ageing treatments. The only answer is to quit.

4. Alcohol

Alcohol is a toxin. It's also a vasodilator, meaning if you drink moderate amounts on a regular basis, the skin feels warm, because your blood vessels actually relax, allowing more blood to flow to the skin. Eventually the blood vessels start to stretch, which leads to greater blood vessel formation, ultimately giving the skin a ruddy look. Alcohol also leeches your skin of vitamins and nutrients and impairs the cleansing capability of the liver. If your liver isn't flushing out toxins, your skin will start looking sallow.

Parole points: Keep your alcohol intake in control. Drink no more than three units a day and have at least two alcohol-free days a week. To help your liver eliminate toxins, take a milk thistle supplement. Also, the topical application of vitamins, namely antioxidants, can boost the skin's free-radical scavenging power.

5. The Sun

How good your skin looks with the passing years depends more on how well you have protected it from the environment than on genetics. The damaging effects of UV (ultraviolet) light on the skin is well documented. Without adequate protection, the skin, in trying to protect itself, thickens and produces melanin, the pigment that darkens cells. Any pigment change from UVA and UVB light causes premature ageing (as much as 80 per cent) and increases the risk of skin cancer as well as leaving your complexion looking like an old leather handbag.

And sunbeds? They're worse, as they emit concentrated UVA light that penetrates deeper into the skin than the combination of UVA and UVB rays in sunshine.

Parole points: Keep out of the sun as much as possible and wear a sunscreen. Dipping no lower than SPF15 is the best way to ensure a smooth and unmottled complexion now and in later life.

6. Lack of Water

Temporary dehydration, which may arise when flying long haul for instance, is not a massive skin problem. But if you're constantly dehydrated, that's going to affect how your skin looks. If you're lacking in water, your skin is actually going to look older.

Constantly keeping your levels of hydration up, on the other hand, will keep the skin supple. Think of a sponge: when dry it's stiff, when wet it's soft. Skins tissues, protein and collagen are all designed to function best in moist conditions.

Parole points: Waterlog your skin by drinking at least eight glasses of water a day.

 TIME TO DITCH *It doesn't matter how many points you score for good skincare, an uptight lifestyle will equal an uptight skin (usually a dry one).*

CHANGE IT NOW *Chill out your skin, along with yourself, with relaxation treatments like massage.*

A workout for the face

Like the muscles in other parts of your body, the muscles in the face absorb and store a lot of tension. The jaw and facial muscles are also some of the busiest muscles in the body: they open, shut, frown, grimace, chew, speak, laugh and sometimes cry many times a day. With all this facial stress, no wonder there's a rush for Botox jabs to paralyse the wrinkles. But hold the syringe! You can build up the skin with movement and massage instead.

When you have a stiff neck, just think how tense the rest of your body is. It's the same for facial muscles. Unless you relax them, they become hard and strained-looking, making you look older. If your muscles are saggy, so is your skin. It folds and you get crow's feet. Move and massage the skin and you will plump it up, as it will increase circulation to the area and bring much-needed nutrients and oxygen to rejuvenate it. So, flex those fingers and get set for some skin prepping!

Taking a few minutes each day to really massage in your chosen moisturiser or night cream, along with these movements, can be enough to give your complexion some get up and glow.

THE NECK TIGHTENER

To help relieve and prevent a double chin, sit upright, head back, looking at the ceiling with your lips closed, and start a chewing motion. You will feel the muscles working in your neck and throat area. Repeat 20 times.

THE FURROW SMOOTHER

For pesky forehead wrinkles, lift your eyebrows as high as possible, opening your eyes very wide. Relax and repeat 10 times.

Then let your fingertips meet in the centre of your forehead and gently lift up the forehead skin while lowering your eyebrows. At the same time draw your finger across the forehead towards the hairline. Repeat 10 times.

THE LIP PLUMPER

Sit upright, keeping your lips closed and teeth together. Smile as widely as you can without opening your lips. Hold for a count of five and when relaxing start puckering your lips in a pointed kiss. Keep it there for a count of five and relax. Repeat 10 times.

THE CHEEK SHAPER

Smile with your lips closed and then suck in your cheeks towards and onto your teeth. Hold this for 10 counts and repeat 10 times.

THE CHIN FIRMER

Raise your chin up and put your lower lip over your top lip. Place your fingers just above your jawbone. Now smile. You will feel a lift in your neck, jaw, mouth and lower cheeks. Hold for 10 counts and release. Repeat 10 times.

The Eye Debagger

Sit upright with your eyes closed and relaxed. Keeping them closed, lift your eyebrows and stretch your eyelids down as far as possible. Hold this position for a count of five. Repeat five times.

To gently tone the muscles of the eye, press your two index fingers on each side of your head at the temples while opening and closing your eyes quickly. Repeat five times.

GET GORGEOUS: 20 INSTANT MAKEOVER SKIN TIPS

1. Keep your eye make-up remover in the fridge. The coolness will stimulate the eye area and help reduce dark circles and puffiness.

2. Try and sleep on your back. It will help with natural drainage and you'll rise with no sleep wrinkles and skin that looks rested and younger.

3. Blemishes form due to unwanted bacteria and zinc plays a key anti-bacterial role in the immune system, so zinc-rich foods equal fewer spots. Find zinc in steak, wheatgerm and Brazil nuts or take an RDA of 15mg in supplement form.

4. Another easy exercise for a fitter face is to mouth the letters 'I', 'E', 'U' and 'X'. Ham it up, exaggerating the pronunciation of each letter so that you feel the muscles really working.

5. As a rescue remedy, apply a tiny bit of haemorrhoid cream onto the orbital bone below your eye. It will shrink bags.

6. Blackhead removal strips I hail as I can't-live-without. They're perfect when you haven't got time for a facial.

7. Indulge in a professional facial four times a year, when the seasons change, to reassess your skin's needs. It really makes a difference and keeps your skin on track.

8. Don't sleep with the heating on. It can cause puffiness in the face, especially around the eyes.

9. Cleanse your face before you work out. Moisturiser and make-up seal the skin and block the evaporation of sweat, both of which can lead to suffocated pores.

10. Cut down on your salt. Besides causing puffiness in the face, high iodine intake can trigger breakouts in those who are acne prone.

11. Make love, not wrinkles. Lovemaking boosts hormones that reduce fatty tissue and increase lean muscle. Studies show that those who regularly make love can look up to 12 years younger than their real age.

12. Cleanse with good-quality cotton-wool pads dampened with cold water.

13. Invest in a magnifying mirror so you can see your skin in every little detail.

14. When cleansing, pull your hair right back. It encourages you to deep cleanse the sides of the face and behind the ears – areas that are often neglected.

15. Masks are more penetrating if, after applying them, you cover your face with a clean warm flannel.

16. Swap your dinner date for a lunch date. Around 2 p.m. is when skin naturally looks its best. At that time it is plump with moisture and not producing too much oil.

17. A little piece of light-coloured fluffiness, as in a scarf worn next to your skin, is very flattering.

18. Pinch your skin. If it's slow to snap back, the chances are you're dehydrated and need to glug some H_2O.

19. Keep cleansing wipes by your bed. That way, even after a busy night, you will never forget to remove your make-up.

20. Wake up your skin and get rid of puffiness by pressing your fingertips gently along the bone running under the eye and up to the temples.

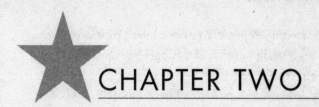 CHAPTER TWO

Shake (and wake) up your make-up

'Beauty, to me, is about being comfortable in your own skin. That or a kick-ass red lipstick.'
Gwyneth Paltrow

The makeover lesson here is about making the most of your face with make-up. Let this chapter act as your in-store beauty consultant, the person you would normally come across at a department store, but minus the hard sell!

Some women say that make-up scares them. They look on in envy as some of their friends expertly achieve that 'no make-up' make-up look from their well-organised make-up bags, while they have spent countless years shopping around for The Eyeshadow, The Lipstick and The Foundation that are going to change their life, or at least their look. Alas, more often than not these very expensive luxuries are never used more than once or twice, with disappointing results, and are left to go rancid on the bathroom shelf.

Some women feel that showing an interest in make-up is

shallow or exercising extraordinary vanity. I don't consider this is the case at all, as a new lipstick or a flush of blush can change your mood as well as knock off years.

Whether it's a case of a lack of confidence or sheer I-can't-be-bothered-ness, you can get over it now! Here I explain what make-up can do for you. Rest assured that make-up help has well and truly arrived.

Are you stuck in a great (big) beauty rut?

Think you can't get stuck in the make-up land that time forgot? Well, think again. I have written about beauty for over ten years and pride myself on being up to speed on everything that sells on a counter near you. I was the last person I (smugly) thought would be stuck in a rut. How misguided I was. On a photographic shoot I recently told a make-up artist I didn't suit red lipstick. 'Nonsense,' she said. 'You're just used to wearing a neutral gloss and you're lacking the confidence to pull it off.' Which got me thinking. Perhaps I had got stuck in a rut but never realised it. I promptly headed off to the nearest department store and lip tested some vibrant hues. The reaction was amazing. My husband asked me if some guy had taken me out for lunch that day. And over cocktails my girlfriends were all asking for the shade and rethinking their make-up.

And let me let you into another secret about the power of lipstick: research shows women who wear it kiss their partners more often than women who don't! And they also tend to enjoy more active social lives.

Old make-up habits can die hard, so how can you tell if

you're stuck in a rut? Apart from the obvious – the same can-do-it-with-my-eyes-shut make-up routine every single day for the past however many years regardless of the occasion – there are other clues.

If all the colours in your make-up bag are a variation on a theme – say, brown – that's classed as a rut in my books. And if you're still feverishly looking for products that were discontinued a while ago, that's a rut too. There's a good reason why products are phased out: textures and colours change. You probably wouldn't be looking for the exact tiered skirt you were wearing years ago, would you, so why the same colour eyeshadow?

And take a moment to question why make-up houses bring out seasonal colours. No, not just to make you spend money – although of course that's their aim – but because skin tone and texture change seasonally and colour and formulations should ideally move along too. The biggest rut you can fall into when it comes to make-up is being scared of change.

The 10 Big Beauty Ruts (to dig yourself out of)

1. You view shopping for make-up as a chore rather than a joy.
2. Your foundation is panstick (very, very thick).
3. Your concealer highlights rather than hides your flaws.
4. There's a bold orange strip running from your cheek to your jaw.
5. Your make-up glitters rather than shimmers.

6. Your black eyeliner makes your eyes appear harsh instead of smoky.
7. Your lipliner shouts 'Hello!' before you do.
8. Your eyelashes look clogged rather than 'volumised'.
9. 'Frost' describes the texture of your make-up rather than a weather condition.
10. Your neck is wearing foundation.

Making over (or under) your make-up bag

A grubby over-stuffed make-up bag is a beauty hazard. But many of us have cosmetic separation anxiety when it comes to our make-up bags. We're loath to let go of old beauty products. Nevertheless, detoxing your bag is the first step towards making over your look. Most importantly, it frees up your time – looking for your keys is bad enough in the morning, let alone a concealer and lipstick – plus it gives you the opportunity to chuck out stuff that's past its sell-by-date and the excuse to go shopping.

When They're Ready to Go

We are all too aware of the fact that beauty isn't eternal – and neither are the products. Here's when to ditch them.

Mascara: Replace it every three or four months. Wait any longer and eye-irritating bacteria may begin to breed. If you have an eye infection, toss your mascara straight away.

Eyeshadows: Depending on how they're stored, creams

can last a year or two, powders longer, since they don't oxidise or contain water. If they develop a cakey top layer, scrape the surface with a butter knife to reveal fresh colour.

Lipstick: Made of wax, it lasts for years, although heat can cause a change in its consistency, colour and texture.

Foundation: It should last a year providing you have stored it in a cool place and kept the lid tightly sealed. If it thickens, separates or smells bad, then toss it.

Face powder: Should last two years, although if stored in the steamy air of a bathroom it can become damp and cloggy. Keep it 'powdery' and fairy-dust light by storing it elsewhere.

Lip and eye pencils: These keep about two years as long as you keep them out of the sun, as waxes will obviously melt.

Brushes: Dirty brushes could be the reason why your make-up doesn't look as good as it should. They can also be the main cause of skin irritation as the result of bacteria and stale sebum hanging about on them. Clean them every week – more often in summer – by washing them in warm water with a little mild shampoo. Then rinse them until the water runs clear. Reshape them and lay them flat on a tissue to dry naturally. Your look will stay fresher for it.

ORGANISING YOUR COMPLETE MAKE-UP KIT

If there's one thing on a shoot that the models and I tend to gravitate towards, it's the make-up artist's cosmetics box. It's fascinating. It's usually a Pandora's box full of exciting colour and lovely packaging and the organisation that goes into it is second to none.

First off, it's never a bag, it's a travel case with tiered pull-out drawers or trays. You can find them in department stores. Secondly, the products are grouped in each drawer, so there are no lipsticks cohabiting with mascaras and such like. And make-up artists are meticulous about putting everything back in its correct place straight after they've used it. This way beauty buys are well looked after, last longer and aren't forgotten.

 TIME TO DITCH *Your yearly make-up bag clearout.*

CHANGE IT NOW *Detox every month. And invest in a clear make-up bag – this way you automatically clean it up when it first begins to look grubby.*

Professional make-up artists say the way you store your beauty booty should reflect the way you apply your make-up. So, layering your case from the base upwards, put foundations and nail polishes at the bottom of the case, keeping bottles upright and lids screwed on tight. This way air cannot get in, risking a change of formulation, and liquids won't pour out too quickly when opened. Bulky items such as compacts or face powders can also be put here. In the next tray or compartment place eyeshadows and blushers. Keep all make-up brushes in a small pencil case so they stay tidy, clean and in shape. In the top section keep lipsticks (for quick reference store them upside down so you can see the shade label), balms, tweezers, eye pencils, mascara and concealer. If you're in a hurry these are always the make-up staples you grab first to make you look presentable in double-quick time.

 TIME TO DITCH *Gunky bottle tops that prevent make-up lids from screwing on tightly.*

 CHANGE IT NOW *Keep baby wipes in your make-up kit to wipe around the tops of bottles after use.*

THE MAKE-UP MUST HAVES

'Use a make-up table with everything close at hand and don't rush, otherwise you'll look like a patchwork quilt.'

Lucille Ball

These must haves are what I class as the desert island essentials. Individually, you wouldn't say any have the 'wow' factor and they may even sound a little obvious and boring. But you'll be surprised how many women don't actually have any of these things in their make-up bags. And they can all be 30-second ways to glamorise your look.

Once you have acquired these basics then you can start to build up your make-up collection by introducing seasonal colours or palettes for a more daring you.

I have purposely not branded these buys either by name or colour, as there are no universal colours or textures to suit absolutely everybody's taste or skin tone. It's up to you to experiment!

The Top Five Make-Up Bag Essentials

★ *A do-it-all sheer foundation:* That's one that's light reflective with antioxidants and an SPF. They're ultra-blendable and give skin a flawless younger finish.

★ *A state-of-the-art concealer:* Look for a liquid one to apply under the eyes with specially treated pigments to lighten shadows along with optical diffusers that help blur lines. Apply sparingly, so it's easier to blend. For blemishes go for a cream concealer which you can 'spot' blend on troubled areas.

★ *Translucent powder:* Dusting powder on over your foundation or just on its own will give your face a smooth and 'rested' appearance. It will also hold your concealer in place. Use with a professional velour puff – one that's generous in size. Buy separately if necessary.

★ *Cream blusher:* I recommend cream that you can dab and blend on and out with fingertips, as I believe it gives that locked-in glow much better than blushing up with powder. The subtle light reflection a cream gives makes for a healthier and dewier look.

★ *Black mascara:* Bat them, flutter them and flirt with them, but never leave lashes naked of mascara. Mascara is the best seduction weapon you'll ever have!

THE ESSENTIAL EXTRAS

Bronzing powder: Perks up a pale complexion. And a sun-kissed look can come across as simply irresistible. Bronzing powder makes the skin look alive and should be dusted over bony areas where the sun hits first: nose, forehead and cheekbones.

Eyelash curlers: The saviour of many a straight lash. Clamping and curling the lashes instantly opens up the whole eye.

Lengthening mascara: For everyday use, this kind of mascara will go on evenly and look very natural. To plump up skinny lashes, opt for a thickening mascara.

Black or brown eyeliner: Apply well and it draws people to your gaze. Simply smudge into top lash lines then wrap under the lower lashes and blend out for wide-eyed appeal.

An iridescent white eyeshadow: Used as a highlighter on the browbone, it works as a wake-up call for tired eyes. The light, pearly pigments brighten eyes on contact.

A neutral powder eyeshadow: Taupe, slate, chocolate brown ... choose two or three 'safe' colours that you can colour sweep over the entire eyelid. You can then build on this collection and add 'fashion' colours such as silvers, blues or pale greens when the occasion suits.

Slanted tweezers: Even the tiniest of hairs will have trouble escaping slanted tweezers!

Brow pencil: Instantly gives shape and definition to sparse brows.

An easy-to-use lip-toned sheer lipstick: Meet your new best friend. Even when you haven't a mirror it's fool-proof to apply and delivers a just-bitten-your-lip transparent stain. Plus if you decide to apply lip colour, it won't creep into fine lines around the mouth.

A lush-coloured lipstick: A highly pigmented colour gives drama to the lip.

Vaseline: A little pot that can multi-task. Slick it onto lips or eyebrows and even rub it into your cuticles.

BRUSHING UP

Although the skill of fingertips shouldn't be under-estimated when applying make-up, it's brushes that are seen as the tools of the trade. And they aren't to be skimped on. Buy the best you can, as good-quality hair can make all the difference to your make-up application.

Brushes

Eyes: To lay down an even layer of shadow, a full soft brush works best. A brush with short bristles is good for applying colour in the crease and outer corners of the eye. Lining the eye relies on a thin, stiff brush.

Eyebrows: I find the best brush to tidy brows is spiral and firm, just like a mini loo brush. It expertly pushes every hair into place.

Face: If not using a velour puff, a large soft brush with a tapered shape is best, since bristles of different lengths can follow the curves around the nose, chin and mouth.

Cheeks: A blush brush should be smaller than a powder brush and should be soft and plush.

Lips: A stiff brush is key. Too soft and the brush will fan out and lose control of the colour. The brush tip should be slanted but not too short otherwise the colour cannot be painted on evenly.

Your make-up master class

For some women a session with a professional make-up artist would be their idea of beauty bliss, as you can learn how to put a great look together in under half an hour (any longer and you're trying too hard!) For others it might be a beauty nightmare. But whatever your feelings, a little knowledge goes a long way...

I always used to be make-up shy until I started writing about beauty. I wore a naked face for years. It wasn't until I started cross-examining make-up artists and watching them in action that I realised what I was missing out on. What difference mascara makes! How much plumper lips look when glossed over! How passionate the complexion looks when flushed with blush! Now I can't look at somebody without wanting to take tweezers to their unruly eyebrows, as I know it would make such a big improvement to their look. Plus I learned it takes a lot of skill and savvy to achieve that elusive no make-up make-up look.

Understandably, you may be wary when seeking the help of a make-up artist at a salon or store. It's not uncommon to be worried that you will be sucked into adopting a look you don't necessarily like or think is you. The most impartial teachers (who have no vested interest in getting you to buy specific products or brands) tend to be professionals who ordinarily work with models or actresses on shoots or sets and charge very generously for their services outside that arena. Although no make-up artist myself, I have been privileged to work with some of the best in the business, and through just sitting back and observing you can learn an awful lot. In fact one of the most invaluable lessons is learning what you can do without rather than what to add – a makeunder rather than a makeover. Here are some other tips I've picked up.

 TIME TO DITCH *The red-eyed bunny look after removing make-up.*

CHANGE IT NOW *For weary-looking eyes, put witch hazel in the fridge, then soak cotton wool pads in it and place them on your eyelids for ten minutes.*

HOW TO DO A FLAWLESS FOUNDATION

The ideal foundation should appear invisible, feel weightless and do amazing things for your complexion. But even with colour choices expanding, making a perfect choice is no easy feat.

Listen up, every woman should have at least two different foundations: one that matches their skin tone in summer and one that flatters a paler skin tone in winter.

Whatever the season, never test foundation on your hand. Test it where you will wear it – simply apply a stripe of it down the middle of your cheek. You'll know when you've come across the right shade, as it will literally disappear into your skin. Check it in natural daylight as opposed to fluorescent light too. If you are still confused about your colour match, seek help from leading firms (Lancôme, Clinique and Elizabeth Arden among others), all of which offer 'customised' foundation services.

Next, application. There's nothing worse than a foundation that looks like it's been laid down with a trowel. Less is more. With your fingertips, apply a little foundation to areas that look uneven or blotchy– maybe the cheeks, the forehead or the sides of the nose. You can always add more if need be. Using your fingertips will warm the foundation, making it like a second skin. Blend it away into 'nothingness'.

If you don't like to wear foundation, go for a tinted moisturiser. If you require more coverage, opt for a liquid, cream or cream-to-powder one. For an oily complexion it makes sense to go with an oil-free formula.

HOW TO DO CLEVER CONCEALER

Like foundation, you require two concealers: one for under the eyes (a light-textured yellow-based one to take away the blue tones) and a thicker match-your-skin-tone shade for blemishes.

When applying concealer under the eye, mix it with a little eye cream so it doesn't cake on, and for spots or redness, use a cotton bud for precise application and blend it around the edges with your fingertips. Remember, you don't want concealer to be too sheer, as it won't disguise what it's supposed to be disguising.

Finish with a fine dusting of loose translucent powder all over.

HOW TO DO GORGEOUS BLUSH

The idea with blush is that it should mimic that lovely flush you get when you've been up to something that's pleasurable! Call it a post-lovemaking glow.

Personally, I'm a lover of cream blush. The right shade and texture can whip up a clean and fresh flush, plus they blend most easily into the cheeks.

Sheer formulations and a well-judged hand are essential. To blush with style and not embarrassment, start with the tiniest of dabs on the apples of the cheeks, then blend the blush up and out towards the temples.

If you have oily skin, however, a cream will not be ideal, as it won't sit well on the skin. A powder blush will suit your skin type best. Dip your brush into the powder and swirl it in circular motions on the apples of your cheeks.

As for colour, generally women with fair to medium skin blush best with corals and transparent pinks, and olive and dark-skinned women should go for shades at the orange end of the spectrum.

As for bronzer, dust colour onto the temples, the bridge of the nose and the chin to capture a natural sun-kissed look rather than a contrived product-developed effect.

HOW TO DO A SEXY SMOKY EYE

Cleopatra had this down to a fine art form, but for the rest of us, black eyeliner and shadow (the beauty equivalent of the little black dress) can be hard to handle. Super-dark shades can make eyes look smaller and closer set. So what's the secret of getting it right?

Essentially, it's taking your time. Make-up artists spend the most time playing up and working on the eyes, as it takes a certain amount of know-how and concentration. Ultimately, you want people to look at your eyes, not your make-up.

For best results, use a charcoal, silver or slate grey powder eyeshadow and take the colour up to the eye socket, blending it into the crease. Then take colour close to the upper lashes and wrap it along and under the lower lash line. Smudge out either with a ring finger or a cotton bud. There should be no harsh lines anywhere. To make eyes really 'pop', apply a light-coloured shimmery shadow right under your eyebrow along the brow bone.

Next: liner. Liquid liners are not foolproof, so it's best to go for an eyeliner pencil that gives the softest finish and is easy to handle. Hold the eyelid taut by pulling the skin up from the temple and dot to dot the pencil along the base of the lashes, then fill in between.

Apply mascara by holding it horizontally and slowly twirl the brush as you move it from the lash root up to and beyond the tips.

HOW TO DO A BRIGHT EYE

Sparkling emerald greens and Mediterranean blues give the element of surprise when colourwashed over the lid. The secret to pulling off and 'grounding' these vivid colours is taming the overall look with a dark eyeliner pencil. This makes them easy and less shockable to wear. The finished look should be smudgy and not precise. Colour should only be applied up to the eye socket, never to the browbone, and the upper and lower lashes should be lined with pencil. If going for this look, keep the rest of the face quiet.

HOW TO DO GREAT LASHES

Eyelashes tend to look thickest and most luxurious between the ages of five and fifteen. That's why mascara was invented! High-tech formulas and perfectly engineered bristles can do so much for the lashes – one brush can totally change the look of the eye.

Here's how to brush with greatness for whatever look you're after:

★ *Thickness:* The more mascara you apply, the thicker your lashes will look. Gently wedge the brush into the base of the lashes and pull it up and out. Comb the lashes between each coat. Just be sure to add extra coats while the first one is still wet to stop it from looking flaky.

★ *Lengthening:* Apply two coats of mascara, combing the lashes in between each coat. While they are still wet, just play up their outer corner by swiping them with the brush.

★ *Volume:* To boost up lashes, simply wiggle the wand along the base of the lash line before drawing it out.

★ *Natural:* If lashes are light, use a dark brown mascara rather than a black one. Before applying it, wipe the wand with a tissue. Brush on only one coat.

HOW TO DO WELL-ARCHED BROWS

I cannot stress enough the importance of eyebrows. Unruly brows have the unflattering effect of dragging the face down and making you look miserable. But as well as framing the face, well-plucked brows are an effortless way to appear more polished and even younger. No kidding!

Like everything else, brows go through fashion phases, thick or thin, but personally I believe you should stick with a shape that suits your face. Now for the perfect pluck plan – but please say and do only when sober!

If you are uncertain about getting the right shape, see an expert (ask in beauty spas and department stores) who will do the job for you. Then you can maintain the shape at home.

When tweezing, be sure not to overpluck. Tweeze rebel hairs between the brows and below the browbones. For the tops of the brows, brush brows straight up, press the brush over the brows and use a pair of small nail scissors to trim any hairs that peek over it. Step back from the mirror every few hairs to check your handywork from a distance.

Fill in brows with a pencil or shadow in the same shade as your base hair colour.

For brow setting, you can either slick over a small amount of Vaseline or use a clear brow gel.

Tweeze stray hairs every two or three days to keep brows in constant shape. I always keep a pair of tweezers near my toothbrush along with a small compact mirror so I don't forget.

HOW TO DO A RED LIP

'Hand me my purse, will you, darling? A girl can't read that sort of thing without her lipstick.'

Audrey Hepburn as Holly Golightly in Breakfast at Tiffany's

The moral of the tale for brightening your lip is: Don't be afraid to try something new — even if you don't think it will suit you!

If the intensity of red scares you, wear it as a tint, balm or gloss rather than an intense matt finish. This will give a mild-mannered ruby red stain. Simply slick it on and blend it in with your fingertip.

Applying a scarlet lipstick from the bullet takes a bit more groundwork. To prep the lips, start off by applying a little lip balm. Then line the lips with a lip pencil in a shade complementary to your lipstick shade. I don't need to remind you that two-tone lips are a definite no-no! Stretch your mouth out into a big smile and follow the natural line of your lips. Then take a lip brush, pick up colour from the lipstick bullet and brush it on. Apply several layers, blotting with tissue paper in-between coats.

As a colour check, take note that blue-reds generally look best on fair skin, warm orange-reds on olive complexions and deep pink-reds on a dark skin.

When wearing red lips it's wise to play down the blush. You don't want to look overheated.

 TIME TO DITCH *A flat-looking skin.*

CHANGE IT NOW *For the most gorgeous glow, mix one third liquid bronzer with two thirds foundation and apply the mixture to your complexion.*

HOW TO DO EVENING MAKE-UP

First, don't panic! Taking your make-up from the desk to dinner to the dance floor can take just 15 minutes.

To begin with, there's no need to completely redo your foundation. The secret is to even out your complexion rather than layering it with yet more products. Mop up excess facial oil with blotting paper (keep it in your desk drawer) and then dab on your concealer(s) to clean up the skin. Lightly pat and blend them out to into red areas, blemishes and under the eyes.

To add vibrancy to the face you want a product that delivers a shimmer. And for that you need a highlighter that cleverly adds dimension to the face. Pat a tiny bit of highlighter along your browbone and with your fingertips feel your cheekbones and highlight the tops to mimic the reflection of light onto the face.

If your eyes are feeling a little computer sore, wake them up with the sparing use of eye drops. Then apply a very pale pink creamy pencil to the inner and outer corner of each eye and watch them instantly perk up.

For lips, dab a spot of highlighter on your cupid's bow (the 'V' at the centre of your top lip) for a natural-looking plumping effect. For dressing up your lips, never apply new colour over old. It can congeal and look messy. Apply lip balm, run a damp tissue gently back and forth across the lip to remove old colour and any dead skin and then decide whether to go for a just-bitten-your-lip shade or something a little stronger and sexier.

Make-Up for your Decade

★ *Twenties:* Treatment foundations can be key to your look, especially if you're suffering from breakouts. Lips will be at their fullest, so take advantage of that lovely pout by seeking out exciting lip colours.

★ *Thirties:* The hectic decade. Skin can lack lustre, so play it up with light-reflecting foundations and carefully appointed highlighters. Multi-sticks can be invaluable to inject life into cheeks, lips and eyes in seconds.

★ *Forties:* The right foundation and concealer are important, as skin will demand more coverage. But keep them light. Too thick and they will begin to look like Polyfilla. Wearing blush will bring back a youthful glow.

★ *Fifties and beyond:* Skin tone will start to fade and eyebrows and lashes will begin to look sparse. The key word here is *strengthen*. Boost your look by defining lashes and brows and upgrading to a brighter shade of blush to counteract the loss of tone in your skin. You don't want your complexion to look bereaved.

WHY EXPERIMENTING WITH MAKE-UP IS SMART!

★ Because unlike wardrobe and hairstyle changes, make-up changes are easy to make without a big deal debut.

★ Because compared with clothes, make-up is relatively cheap.

★ Because unlike a haircut, you can wear one colour one
day and a new one the next.

★ And because thanks to the growing number of over-the-
counter samples available, you don't have to buy something to try it.

Many women think experimenting should be reserved just
for the young, but I disagree. You can always try out unexpected colours. Your look shouldn't be bound by years of
tradition; ideally, it should be free-spirited. And whatever
your age, you will always have lots of options to get glamorous.

At the end of the day make-up should be fun, and experimenting can be very uplifting not only for the face but also
for the soul. And it isn't surgery. If you don't like it, wipe it
off and try something else.

A simple change of texture can easily pave the way out of
a beauty rut. Changing the formula, not the colour, of your
staple products is a subtle and effective way to tweak your
look – and it can produce big results. For instance, swap a
compact foundation which can give a flat-looking complexion for a tinted moisturiser that can instantly recreate a
post-gym glow. Or you could upgrade a rosy lipgloss to a
pale pink lipstick, making for a more sophisticated look,
and supercharge a grey powder eyeshadow to a gunmetal
cream shadow. Get the idea? Be inspired to try out new
shades as if you were in a changing room trying on different dresses!

GET GORGEOUS: 20 INSTANT MAKEOVER MAKE-UP TIPS

1. To liven up sleepy eyes extra-fast, colourwash the lid with a coppery cream shadow.
2. Always blush up in natural daylight to avoid cherry jam cheeks.
3. A vibrant pink lip looks amazing against olive skin.
4. Dust a little bronzer under your chin to strengthen up your jawline.
5. After applying lipstick, finish with a dab of gloss in the centre of your bottom lip. It creates a sexy 3D effect.
6. When applying eyeliner, lean your elbow on a hard surface to ensure steadiness.
7. Eyeshadows will crease unless you powder lids first. Translucent powder swept over lids is all you need for a great base.
8. Thin lips will never look thick unless cosmetically plumped up. Refrain from lining over your natural lip line and instead choose a light-toned lipstick and swipe over a touch of shiny gloss.
9. Use a well-sharpened pencil for eyes and a blunter one for lips. There's nothing worse than a hard lip line.
10. Fake the effects of a facial by using a tinted moisturiser. It brightens the whole complexion.
11. If you have small eyes, stay away from dark shades on the inner corner of the eye. Elongate the eye by lining from the outer corner to just three-quarters of the way in.
12. Do your blush and lips first and you'll be less likely to

be heavy-handed when you're applying shadow and liner. It's easy to overdo the eyes when there's no other colour on the face.

13. Lipstick should grow bolder over the years. Neutrals look great on a young skin, but can look washed out on an older skin. From your mid-forties, learn to love colour.

14. If skin is already tanned, drop the bronzer. Why overcook the result?

15. To completely make-up in a minute, choose multi-use sticks where colour works anywhere. Apply to eyes, cheeks and lips for a slightly different but matching effect.

16. To prevent make-up meltdown, invest in an oil-free primer. This initial layer evens out skin texture, ensuring make-up glides on smoothly and doesn't wander.

17. To help a brow pencil glide as opposed to tug, warm the tip by rolling it in between your fingers or giving it a short sharp blast with the hairdryer.

18. If playing up cheeks with a bright blush, use a sheer hue in the same colour family on the lips.

19. If your skin is freckly, don't bury it under a thick layer of foundation. Let the freckles shine through.

20. To be a real eye-opener, experiment with coloured mascaras. Dark maroon shades look great with hazel eyes, emerald green with blue and deep purple with green. Likewise, eyes can also really stand out by lining them with coloured eyeliner.

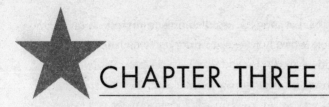

CHAPTER THREE

More than just make-up

'Those who look for beauty find it.'
Unknown

When it comes to looking good, it invariably comes down to all those modest details that never escape the eye. Hands, feet, neck, even elbows and knees are frequently unattended zones but always attract the gaze. Who hasn't looked at a woman's chipped nails or cracked heels and written her off as dishevelled? Even worse, if you're in a position of power it makes you look out of control, so how can you expect others to follow your lead? And be warned: although you can get away with 'shabby chic' when talking interiors, when it comes to personal appearance, a thrown together, crumpled appearance never looks chic and bohemian, just lazy and messy.

The word 'groomed' is rather an old-fashioned term today and whips up the image of brushing and teasing dogs for the judging at Crufts. But nevertheless it's a beauty skill that should never be neglected. It's said that the Duchess of Windsor had all her walls painted the same colour as her face powder so that she would be bathed in gratifying light. Now I'm not suggesting you go to those

great lengths, but often I've watched extreme makeovers on television where women practically remortgage their house for a
facelift and I think, 'If you had your teeth professionally whitened or
realigned with veneers, there'd be no need for the scalpel. Your
bright and sexy smile would lift your face and make you look
radiant.'

Unfortunately only a handful of us will ever be naturally beautiful,
but with a little work and time anyone can look perfectly groomed
and immeasurably improved.

And, as the title of this chapter suggests, it's far more than just
powder and lipstick that makes for an impeccably polished
gorgeousness. It's things like picking a fragrance which makes an
impact the minute you walk into a room. Even making over your
sleeping habits can make a huge difference to the way you look.
A lack of shuteye can accelerate ageing and pile on the pounds,
and a sunken mattress can knock two inches off your height. Not
the recipe for a sleeping let alone a wide-awake beauty! So here's
how to groom yourself for beauty success.

How to play a winning hand

Hands are always on show. We literally talk with them. Think how much you wave them around to express what you are trying to describe. And they reveal all. Your complexion may look one age but your hands quite another!

I think it's ironic that women are so concerned about the ageing of their face that they completely forget about their hands. When all's said and done, they battle the same level of exposure to the elements, so why should their skin age any differently from that on the face? In fact, compared with our complexion, our hands have thinner skin, less wrinkle-and-vein-obscuring fat and fewer moisturising oil glands – an average of only 100 per square inch compared to 900 on the same sized bit of facial skin. This all adds up to the fact that the hands can age far faster than the complexion.

 TIME TO DITCH: *Mottled hands.*

 CHANGE IT NOW: *Wear sunscreen on the backs of your hands. It's one of the most important things you can do for them.*

In dermatologists' offices, treatments for hands are now catching up with those for the face. Laser therapy is zapping broken capillaries, bulging veins are being injected with solutions to collapse them, glycolic acid peels are getting rid of tell-tale sunspots and collagen injections are being used to fatten up the backs of hands which have become thin and bony with the advancing years. There is also a lot you can do for yourself.

Hand-Me-Down Tips for Better Hands

★ Fake tan can give hands a younger appearance.

★ The most common problem for hands is dehydration, so moisturise whenever the thought strikes you. Keep a tube of hand cream at the sink, on your desk and on the bedside table.

★ For ageing hands, look for hand creams that contain much the same ingredients as those for the face: sun protection factors, retinol and glycolic acid, for instance.

★ When in the shower, exfoliate the backs of the hands with a body scrub. They will look instantly revitalised.

★ Wear gloves – that's gardening gloves, washing-up gloves, gloves in cold weather and, for the dedicated, even driving gloves. You get a lot of UV exposure through the windscreen.

★ For a surge of intensive moisture, apply a moisture-treatment hand cream and pop on cotton gloves to enhance the effects. You may look like

> Michael Jackson, but hey, it works.
> ★ Alternatively, washing-up can double up as an intensive heat treatment. Apply a hand or face mask, slip on a thin pair of cotton gloves, then don your rubber gloves on top and plunge your hands into hot water.

NAILED! THE SECRETS OF DOING A PROFESSIONAL MANICURE

How well your hands and nails are groomed says a great deal about you as a person. Ragged cuticles throw out the impression you're literally running yourself ragged and since there's nothing difficult about hand and nail care, there's really no excuse for a less than hand(some) pair of hands!

Nail bars are now just as numerous and popular as coffee bars. The concept originated in New York, where manicures are part of many women's weekly routine. And it's little wonder: nail know-how can be your secret beauty weapon. A fresh manicure will accessorise any outfit, quickly lift the spirits and make a sweeping hand gesture a statement in itself.

THE NAILFILE CLINIC

Polish can improve the appearance of nails, but not their health. The condition of your nails runs much deeper than the top layer. To make nails polishworthy, here's a troubleshooting guide to the six most common nail problems.

Weak Nails

Cause: Can result from a lack of proper vitamins and minerals in the diet and overexposure to water and harsh cleaning products

Solution: Check out your diet and apply a penetrating nail hardener weekly. Use an extra-mild polish (acetone free) so as not to further weaken the nails.

Ridged Nails

Cause: Can be hereditary or linked to dermatological disorders as well as illness

Solution: For slightly ridged nails, buff with a specially bought buffer to smooth the surface and give the nails a healthy sheen. Also seek out a specific ridge-filler base-coat treatment.

Bitten Nails

Cause: Low self-esteem, stress, nervousness

Solution: You can use unpleasant polishes that leave a bitter taste, but hardened biters can even begin to like them! Do a weekly manicure, as if nails look attractive it can act as an incentive to stop biting. Keep your hands busy so they're less likely to end up in your mouth.

White Spots

Cause: Most likely to be caused by a blow to the nail plate

Solution: A case of leaving it to grow out. In the interim, disguise with nail polish.

Overgrown Cuticles
Cause: Lack of attention
Solution: Apply cream or oil at least three times a week to keep cuticles soft. Never clip them off.

Discoloured Nails
Cause: Tobacco or the application of dark polishes minus a base coat
Solution: Regular buffing can reduce the discoloration. Or you can try soaking them in a cup of white vinegar every month. Always use a base coat.

A SELF-MADE MANICURE

A manicure is much more than a change of polish, it's one of the best treats you can give yourself. A home manicure should be done once a week and as a rule varnish should only by left on fingernails for six days. You should then have a day without polish to 'air' the nails and then reapply polish the following day.

Cuticle cream or oil should be massaged into the cuticle daily (leave it by your bed) and cuticle remover should only be used once a month.

How do you choose a nail enamel? First, look at the colour, then the price, then the brand. And then what?

First: Clean and Shape
★ Remove any old polish by holding a cotton pad soaked with nail polish remover firmly against the nail for a few

seconds. Wipe off with a single stroke. Remove stubborn polish around the cuticles with a cotton bud dipped in remover.

★ Shape the nails with an emery board. Keep the length short, rounded and just peeking above the finger pad. File in one direction only using long light strokes, a bit like playing a violin. This should prevent friction and heat that will split the nail tip. Avoid filing deep into the corners of the nails. Finish by using gentle downward strokes at the very tip in order to seal the nail layers together.

Next: Soak and Soften

★ You can then add some nail-whitening tablets to warm water and dip and soak your fingers in it for a few minutes. Dry them off and apply cuticle remover around the nail contour. Gently roll back the skin with a cuticle stick, using tiny circular movements all around the nail plate to form a neat outline.

★ Using a cotton bud dipped in nailpolish remover, gently wipe excess oil from the nail plate and under the nail tip.

Finally: Prep and Polish

★ Brush on a good-quality base coat over the entire nail, stopping short of the cuticle. Leave it to dry for a few minutes. It will remain slightly tacky to the touch. This enables the polish to stick better.

★ For the classiest paint job, roll the bottle of varnish between the palms of your hands before using it. Shaking will only trap air bubbles. Apply in two or three thin coats, sweeping the brush around the area of the cuticle and down the middle of the nail, then stroking either side for professional results. If colour floods over the cuticle or seeps around the sides of the nail, either use a corrector pen or dip a cotton bud into remover to clean it off.

★ To stop chipping, act as a colour fix and deliver extra shine, apply a top coat.

★ Leave nails to dry. Do not plunge them into hot water for at least two hours. Water can get under the polish and peel it back.

 TIME TO DITCH *Fashion-dictated nail shapes.*

 CHANGE IT NOW *File your nails so they mirror your cuticle shape, usually an oval. This looks natural and modern.*

Sole diva: your ready-to-wear step class

Would you feel confident enough right this minute to boldly kick off your shoes and bare your soles? Thought not.

There's little doubt that feet are the unsung heroes of the body. But however hardworking they are, they should never look it. Feet *can* look beautiful but most of us leave them to look after themselves, hence multiple corns, ingrowing toenails and hard patches of skin. And a pedicure is more often than not regarded as a luxury, not an essential beauty ritual. One podiatrist tells me some women only come regularly if they have a partner who loves stroking their feet!

GIVE YOURSELF A SOLE REVIVAL

It's a fact that women suffer more foot problems than men and that's not surprising when most of us suffer from shoe vanity – that's choosing a shoe size that's too small and squeezing our feet into pointy toes and heels higher than a New York skyscraper to lengthen the look of our legs. But let's get real: what woman is going to swap her heels for matronly flats in order to save her feet? It goes without saying that fashion overrules foot health most of the time.

I personally think a divine shoe deserves a foot to be proud of. There's nothing worse than slipping off an expensive shoe to reveal a second-rate foot. If your feet are well cared for, you'll walk taller, lighter and straighter too. And there's nothing less attractive than a woman who hobbles!

The way to go for sandal-ready feet all year round is the smart marrying of a podiatrist with a pedicure. A podiatrist will tell you that the people with the best feet don't wear shoes at all – and when you think that feet can live squashed up in shoes 16 hours a day, it's of little surprise that they start to react and develop minor ailments.

To start your makeover on the right foot, here are steps to overcoming the most common foot complaints.

Blisters

Cause: Accumulation of fluid between the skin's inner and outer layers caused by lengthy friction with socks and shoes. Rarely serious, but can become infected if not treated properly.

Solution: Do not burst if possible. However, if they do break, swab them with an antiseptic solution and cover them with a plaster.

Bunions

Cause: These are usually hereditary, but wearing ill-fitting shoes exacerbates the problem. When the big toe that usually points forward curves towards the other toes, this can affect the performance and appearance of other toes.

Solution: To prevent a bunion from becoming worse, wear shoes with a straight inside edge (that's no pointy shoes) to reduce pressure on the joint. A podiatrist may recommend protective pads, shoe alterations or in advanced cases surgery, which is usually successful.

Calluses

Cause: The skin on the foot is four times thicker than anywhere else on the body. In simple terms, calluses are extended areas of thickened skin.

Solution: Two words: exfoliate and moisturise. Gently rub with a pumice stone every day and then slather on an enriched foot cream. If neglected, calluses can become painful and will require treatment with padding.

Corns

Cause: These are small areas of thick tough skin which arise as a result of friction with shoes or from the build up of moisture.

Solution: Do not dig them out yourself or use commercially available cures without professional advice, as these may damage the healthy skin around the corn. Instead see a podiatrist to have them cut out. Try and wear shoes for the majority of the time that let toes 'wiggle'.

Fungal Infections

Cause: Fungal infections are caused by a number of

different organisms. They give rise to itching between the toes, along with red and raw-looking skin. Toenails can become thickened or sore.
Solution: Prevent with good hygiene. Always wash and dry your feet well. Once infected, the skin is relatively simple to treat with creams or powders. The nails, however, can be more difficult to treat. To ensure the most effective treatment, see a podiatrist.

FOR BAREFOOT CHIC

★ Examine your feet daily after bathing when the skin is clean and soft.

★ Trim toenails regularly, at least once a month. Cut straight across to prevent the curving corners that can cause ingrowing toenails.

★ Foot models slather their feet in rich moisture lotion and pop on cotton socks overnight. Why not try it?

★ Exercise your feet daily. Try rising on tiptoes to help strengthen the foot muscles, walking on the outer edges of the feet to tone up the outer arch, rotating the ankles for good circulation and bending the toes downwards as far as possible to strengthen up the muscles in the front of the foot.

A DIY PEDICURE

I think a pedicure is one of the best things you can do for yourself on a Sunday afternoon. It feels luxurious, it's pleasurable and the results are pure foot fetish!

First: Plunge and Pamper

★ Remove any polish from your nails using the same technique as you would for a manicure (*see page 67*). Then soak your feet in a footbath for 10 minutes. Add either essential oils such as lavender or a pre-bought foot soak.

★ To loosen dead skin and help circulation, massage your feet with an exfoliating foot scrub. Opt for creams with an AHA that work harder to leave your feet smoother.

★ When your feet are dry, follow up with a final buffing of hard surfaces with a foot file. Slather on foot lotion.

★ Apply cuticle cream to all around the nail area and leave it to nourish your feet. You may want to use a cuticle exfoliating treatment, as toe cuticles can become hard and dry in shoes and boots. Now gently push back the cuticles with an orange stick wrapped in cotton wool or a nail hoof, using tiny circular movements around the nail plate. Run the orange stick under the nail to get rid of any dirt.

Next: Clip and File

★ Using clippers strong enough to handle the thickness of the nail, clip the nails straight across. 'Bevel' the edge with an emery board. There's nothing more annoying than a rough nail causing a ladder in fine denier tights.

★ Now get rid of those ridges with a buffer.

Finally: Polish and Paint

★ Paint on a good-quality base coat to smooth out the surface and give the polish staying power.

★ If your toes are overlapping, use a toe separator to guarantee a non-smudge paint job. When painting, put your foot up on a higher surface so you can see what you are doing and work from the little toe inwards to avoid knocking the fresh wet polish.

★ Apply two coats of polish as you would for a manicure and finish off with a top coat for protection and high shine. In summer use a top coat with UV protection to stop the nails from yellowing. Never paint nails before bedtime, even the layering of a sheet can cause smudging.

 TIME TO DITCH *The belief that your feet aren't sexy.*

 CHANGE IT NOW *Wear shoes with ankle straps and see how sexy they look and feel.*

How to make over your smile

I hazard a guess that you spent longer drinking your cup of coffee this morning than you did brushing your teeth. The average person only spends 30 seconds brushing their teeth when dentists recommend two minutes. That extra minute and a half could be all you need to makeover your smile.

A study commissioned a couple of years ago highlighted the fact that two thirds of people subconsciously draw negative assumptions about a person's professional status and love lives based on the colour of their teeth. When shown a picture of a woman with stained teeth, only a third of men considered the smile to be an attractive feature. However, almost half of those shown a picture of a person with a sincere white smile voted this a big turn-on.

The smile, when beaming bright, can make more of an impact than a clear complexion. American research shows that a person's teeth and smile are what 63 per cent of us notice first. A leading dentist has even gone as far as to predict that a great smile and good teeth will be the ultimate accessory for the 21st century and without them the chances of success in love, life and business will be limited.

The first step to making your smile that little bit brighter can be carried out right in your bathroom. With your tooth-brush. Brushing your teeth is such a familiar process that it's easy to forget how important it is for the health and look of your teeth.

Become your Own Hygienist

★ **Brush.** There is some evidence that electric tooth-brushes are more effective at removing plaque. Place the brush at the neck of the tooth where it meets the gum and use very short horizontal move-ments at a 45-degree angle to dislodge plaque. If tooth brushing is unhurried, then every surface can be cleaned thoroughly. And change your tooth-brush. This may seem ultra-simple advice, but it's been reported that the average person only buys 1.2 toothbrushes a year even though it's recom-mended that you change your toothbrush every three months.

★ **Floss.** Half of us never floss, yet dental studies show it's the most effective way of shifting plaque and preventing gum disease. Each tooth has five surfaces and brushing only reaches three. The majority of dental disease begins interdentally – that's between the teeth. Toothbrushes cannot reach these spaces, only dental floss can. If your gums bleed slightly, you should continue flossing. The bleeding should stop after a couple of weeks. And remember, nothing ruins your smile faster than a day-old piece of food stuck between your teeth. Yuck!

GETTING A WHITER, BRIGHTER SMILE

I was chatting to a friend of mine but I wasn't really listening to what she was saying, as I was too busy looking at her teeth. They definitely had a 'wow' factor that I had never noticed before. When I asked her about it, she revealed she had forgone her yearly health spa pampering weekend and used the money to get her teeth whitened instead.

We are fast wising up to the fact that whiter teeth make us look healthier and younger. Just as you may have been born with dark hair, so you may have naturally yellow teeth, but just as highlights can lighten your hair colour, so whitening can lighten the colour of your teeth – and it can really make a big difference to your look. In fact, teeth whitening has already become one of the UK's top job perks!

When you think what our teeth encounter over the years – coffee, red wine, coloured foods, cigarettes – it's little wonder that they need a professional whiten now and again. And afterwards your smile feels somehow cleaner, your lipstick looks brighter and you're never afraid to use a big open grin in a photograph again. And whatever your budget there's a method to suit.

Laser Tooth Whitening

This is the most expensive treatment. A non-damaging hydrogen peroxide based gel is applied to the teeth and a laser is used to activate the gel and initiate the whitening process. In just one hour you can whiten your teeth by five shades, although whitening cannot lighten crowns or veneers. Some sensitivity may be experienced for the next day or so.

Dental Tray System

With this method your dentist creates custom-made trays (moulds) for your upper and lower gums that you take home. You then fill them with a bleaching solution and insert them before bedtime for the next two weeks. The gel will sit on your teeth every night and even after a few days they will look considerably whiter. This also gives you control over how white you want your teeth.

Over-the-Counter Tray System

This is the same procedure as the dental tray system, but the gum shields or moulds are not made to measure, so they can be less effective and less comfortable for the wearer. The solution tends to be weaker too.

Whitening Toothpaste

These are more polishing pastes than whitening pastes and can help remove superficial stains. The bleaching agent solution is weak, so don't expect too much.

Doing the White Thing

Keep your teeth looking whiter for longer by:

★ Avoiding eating foods that will stain the teeth. Curry, beetroot and tomato-based sauces are all culprits.

★ Using a straw to drink cola. This way it misses the front of your teeth where staining is most noticeable.

> ★ Cutting down on tea and coffee. They are the worst offenders regarding staining.
> ★ Brushing your teeth after smoking.
> ★ Wearing red lipstick – it will accentuate the whiteness.

MORE WAYS TO IMPROVE YOUR SMILE

Why is it that we are not prepared to put up with a bad hair day, but prepared to put up with bad teeth every day? But if you smile at yourself in the mirror and you don't like what you see, then cosmetic dentistry can give you what nature hasn't. Some refer to it as a 'smile lift'.

Modern dentistry now offers far more than the six-monthly 'fill and drill'. In the fast-paced lucrative world of better-looking teeth, new methods, materials and training are constantly being evaluated, plus it's now socially acceptable to obtain a better-looking smile. It's been said that in five years' time, cosmetic dental surgery will be recognised as better than a traditional facelift, false teeth will be a thing of the past and implants – titanium fixtures anchored into the bone of the jaw – will become more commonplace for people who have lost their teeth.

Three of the Best

Veneers: A thin porcelain or glass-based covering that's permanently bonded over stained, crooked or damaged teeth to give them a perfect appearance. The materials are so good they look completely natural.

Crowns: In the past, crowns often made the teeth look overlarge and the mouth crowded. Today they are modelled by hand and custom-made to mimic the natural teeth in both colour and shape. They fit over teeth that are heavily filled or stained and the latest materials really look like the real thing.

Composite fillings: Instead of showing a mouth full of silver-coloured fillings, you can now have fillings made out of white composite material so the repair is invisible.

Busting your bad beauty habits

'I don't understand how a woman can leave the house without fixing herself up a little. If only out of politeness.'
Coco Chanel

Nobody's perfect – even the best groomed among us have beauty habits we'd rather not share. But what's the point of making yourself over if you're still hanging onto those bad beauty habits that could be jeopardising your look? I've covered picking spots and using dirty make-up brushes already, but believe me there are a whole lot more. Mostly these habits are born out of ignorance rather than idleness, but the outcome is not attractive: infections and spots.

In this rundown of these bad beauty habits, you'll probably recognise a few of your own, so start to kick them out of your routine now.

SHARING MAKE-UP
What's a little lipgloss between friends? A cold sore perhaps! Sharing make-up may be a bonding moment but it can lead to nothing but trouble. It's a terrible practice that can put you on the fast track to eye and skin infections. In

a panic you could borrow powder or blusher, but anything around the eyes or lips should be avoided.

WATERING DOWN COSMETICS

It may be tempting to add a splash of H_2O to your mascara to make it go the extra mile, but apart from unsettling the formulation you could also change the balance of preservatives that keeps make-up safe.

CHEWING YOUR LIP

Not only is this the easiest way to transfer lipstick from your lip to your teeth, but also chewing away on the delicate lip area can trigger bleeding and soreness, leaving the lips red and swollen.

If the habit is linked to nerves, try chewing gum. To solve the problem of flaky chapped lips, use lip balm regularly.

SLEEPING IN YOUR MAKE-UP

You know this is a crime, don't you? The term 'sleep on it' is not meant for foundation and mascara. Apart from ruining a white pillow, fragments of mascara could lodge in the eye. And at night, when skin is renewing itself, stale foundation settles into pores and clogs them, and hey presto, a new breakout.

PEELING OFF NAIL POLISH

This could be a nervous habit, but however relaxing you find it, it isn't pretty! Not only does it look shabby, but the chances are you're scraping your nail away as well, because it's bonded to the varnish. The result will be weakened nails. Always use nail polish remover.

What's giving your age away?

Elbows, knees, neck and décolletage. These are the biggest giveaways of age and prime spots for woeful neglect.

All parts of the body are not created equal. Individual parts need individual attention, but elbows and knees, for instance, are often overlooked. But like the rest of the skin on your body, they are vulnerable to slackening, sun damage and rough texture. Here's how to go from neglect to protect.

ELBOWS

'Give it some elbow grease' is a common phrase and this just indicates how hardworking elbows are. Like feet, they can develop hard skin, and as they are leaned on every day they can soon take on a dingy appearance as dirt becomes ingrained in the skin.

When showering or bathing, exfoliate your elbows along with the rest of your body and moisturise well.

KNEES

Knees look their best between the ages of 15 and 30. After that, they suffer. The constant bending motion causes the skin to sag.

Adding lunges to your exercise routine is said to help tone the knees. Also, because they can develop hard skin ('washer-woman knees'), it's a good idea to buff and moisturise them. They absorb moisture like a sponge, so a great tip is to keep a pot of moisturiser by the loo and rub it into your knees whenever you're sitting on it!

NECK

The neck suffers the same skin enemies as the complexion: gravity, sunlight, smoking and weight loss. Don't wind up with a two-tiered effect – a healthy complexion teamed with a lined turkey-like neck. You only have to extend your routine below the chin and your neck will reap the same anti-ageing benefits as your face.

Repeat after me: 'Bring your skincare down!'

DÉCOLLETAGE

A generous cleavage can look very alluring, but not if it has a crazy paving look due to dehydration and sun damage. Typically, in Europe this area is looked after very well, but in Britain we tend to ignore it.

To protect this area, moisturise to make skin suppler and always use an SPF. If you want to go 'French' about it, look for bust serums or firming bust gels to give you a silicon-free uplift (although don't expect too much!) and an improvement in skin tone. Be aware of spritzing perfume here, as the alcohol content can leave the skin dry.

TIME TO DITCH *Laying bare your décolletage to the sun's rays. It reduces elasticity and can cause the breasts to sag.*

 CHANGE IT NOW *Cover up or make an SPF your new breast friend.*

A pure scent seduction

Let me confess: I find it hard to stay faithful. Before you label me a complete Jezebel, let me assure you I'm talking fragrance. Although it sounds romantic – just think of the association between Marilyn Monroe and Chanel No. 5 – I've never been one to wear a 'signature' fragrance. I'm far too flirtatious when it comes to the olfactory factor and would find it hard sticking with the same scent forever.

Now more than ever fragrance is being worn to reflect our personality and the lifestyles that we lead. Call it 'confidence in a bottle': a global study by a leading cosmetic company revealed that 50 per cent of women said that wearing fragrance made them feel good about themselves.

One of the secrets of why we wear perfume is the complex way certain smells can influence our emotions. Studies have shown that perfume can have a direct effect on the brain via the olfactory nerves and skin absorption. Scientific surveys explain that the most appealing fragrances always bring intense joy to the wearer. But can you honestly say the first scent you fell in love with is the same one you're having a fragranced affair with today? Probably not. The idea of having a lifetime scent is romantic, but in reality would be limiting when there are so many tempting new fragrances launched each year.

'When you say goodbye to your man, you must smell divine – he'll remember your scent all day and not his secretary's.'

ESTÉE LAUDER

You probably have friends, like I do, whose fragrance reaches your nose before they do. I like to call it 'fragrance matchmaking'. So how do you go about finding a scent that makes you memorable?

Today, fragrance is so much more than smelling nice – it's about appealing to your inner image. Just think of the glamorous advertising that is used to convince you that a certain fragrance will make you sexier, slimmer and richer! In essence the 'marketing noses' behind the fragrance want you to say 'That is who I am.'

Although deciding what fragrance to wear has as much to do with the person you want to be as the one you are today, the bottom line is if you don't like the smell, you're not going to buy it. In fact leading fragrance expert Roja Dove goes as far as to say, 'The wrong fragrance on a woman can be as shocking as bright red lipstick on a nun.'

Your beloved fragrance(s) should ideally, with one spritz, blast away jaded spirits and deliver aromatic notes that represent pure escapism. So how do you choose?

quiz

UNLOCK YOUR PERFUME PERSONALITY

Wondering which perfume family suits your personality? Take this ultra-quick quiz to find out.

1. Which colour do you like best?
a) Pink
b) Red
c) Green
d) Chocolate

2. Your dream holiday would be:
a) Paris
b) Thailand
c) Switzerland
d) The Australian outback

3. You overdose on:
a) Cute handbags
b) High-heeled mules
c) Jeans
d) Books

4. How would you describe your style?
a) Very feminine
b) Boho hippy chic

c) The girl next door

d) Classic, but never boring

5. Which beauty treatment is always on your wish list?

a) Manicure

b) Full body massage

c) Facial

d) Reflexology

YOUR SCORE

Mostly As

You're drawn to light and floral fragrances that are relaxed, charmingly sexy and with plenty of personality – just like you! You like a scent that lifts your mood straight away. Sniff out keynotes of rose, orchid, gardenia and sweet pea.

Mostly Bs

You're exotic and sensual and you know how to work your God-given sex appeal to your advantage. Therefore your pulse points will appreciate an opulent and musky oriental scent. Notes of jasmine, ylang ylang, sandalwood and sensual fruit would suit your fragrance personality.

Mostly Cs

You're a free-spirited free-moving social butterfly whose fragrant soul mate is matched in energetic green and citrus notes. As you love the outdoors, a zestful bouquet of grapefruit, lemon, mandarin and orange blossom will get your pulse racing.

Mostly Ds

You're famously grounded and never let your head float too high in the clouds. You know what you like, possess a low-key elegance and have a sensual and earthy nature. You love lingering base notes of cashmere, vetiver and musk against your skin.

★ **TIME TO DITCH** *Smelling like every other woman.*

★ **CHANGE IT NOW** *Wear a man's fragrance.*
Remember, it's only the advertising that stamps the sex on the juice and many scents 'for men' play up perfectly to a woman's pulse points.

Making over your sleep habits

Sleep is more of a beauty treatment than you could ever dream of. Weight gain, red eyes and wrinkles can all be brought on by not enough time spent between the sheets. Good-quality shuteye is the best thing for feeling healthy, looking good and being happy. In fact sleep is essential.

It used to be a badge of honour to say you could party all night, but more of us are now waking up to the fact that sleep is a luxury we can't afford to skimp on. But according to the Sleep Council, it's a luxury that many of us are missing out on, with reports that a large proportion of us are suffering from a severe lack of sleep. With research from the University of Chicago showing that sleeping less than four hours a night for a week causes changes that mimic many of the hallmarks of advanced ageing, perhaps it's a problem you would like to wake up to.

Five Signs You're Sleep Deprived

1. You can't even function until you have had a caffeine fix.

> **2.** The minute you sit down you feel like nodding off.
>
> **3.** You regularly remember your dreams. This indicates that you are waking up before the final sleep cycle – the one where you get the most mind-clearing sleep.
>
> **4.** You can't get up without the shrill bell of an alarm clock. If you've had your quota of restorative sleep, your internal clock should stir on its own.
>
> **5.** You're irritable. Very irritable.

There are several reasons why many of us struggle to sleep the full eight hours, and burning the candles at both ends seems to be one of them. Often this means that we have insufficient time for sleep, or are so stressed that by the time we hit the pillow we can't sleep. Ultimately sleep seems to take a back seat to our social life, work, exercise, television and the internet, leaving us walking around in a chronic state of sleep deprivation.

According to the British Sleep Foundation, for the average person, who needs eight hours' sleep a night, losing even one hour can lower the IQ by one point the next day. This may not sound a lot, but add it up over a week and low-grade absent-mindedness can soon set in.

Now let's talk weight gain. Nutritionists believe that grabbing too little sleep alters our metabolism so our bodies cannot process food effectively. It's claimed that an extra hour of sleep a night can lead to visible weight loss within weeks. This may seem a claim too far, but you know that if you're tired the first thing you reach for is a comforting bar of chocolate and if you stay up late there's always another snack to be had.

IN SEARCH OF A GOOD NIGHT'S SLEEP (MINUS COUNTING SHEEP)

★ Set up a sleep sanctuary. Making your night-time environment conducive to sleep will help your brain recharge. Curl up under a pink duvet or wear pink pyjamas – pink is one of the most restful colours for the bedroom.

★ Peel a banana. High in the amino-acid tryptophan, it helps to promote sleep.

★ Buy a king-size bed. It's a Hollywood myth that you should sleep wrapped in your lover's arms. The only sense you have of your partner while you're in a state of unconsciousness is if they disturb you.

★ Wear socks. If your core body temperature isn't right, you can't sleep. Cashmere socks feel indulgent.

★ Stay away from stimulants for three hours before bed. That's bacon, cheese, chocolate, red wine and horror films!

★ Worry early. Plan your next day early in the evening. This way you won't worry while trying to get to sleep.

★ Dim the lights. Avoid bright lights around the house before bed.

★ Make peace. Never go to bed on a row. Anger is a destructive emotion and prevents you from sleeping.

★ Don't use your bed for anything but sleep and sex. Paying your bills or doing your paperwork in it will make you associate it with wakeful duties.

★ We grow about three-quarters of an inches in the night

(during the day the spine is compressed), so do the Goldilocks thing and invest in a good mattress – one that is neither too soft nor too hard. This will not only ensure a better night's sleep but also give you added height in the morning.

★ Play mind games. Exhaust your brain until it wants to switch off. Play alphabet games such as famous names with double initials, for instance Brigitte Bardot, Charlie Chaplin, Doris Day … get the idea?

GET GORGEOUS: 20 INSTANT MORE THAN MAKE-UP TIPS

1. Bleach dirty elbows back to milky whiteness by cutting a lemon in half and rubbing it deep into the skin.

2. Look for a night cream boasting the herb valerian. It's a natural sleep promoter.

3. If you're having a good day, wear your favourite scent. If you're expecting a bad day, wear it too. You will link that smell with those good memories and it will make you feel better!

4. No time to brush your teeth after a meal? Sugarless gum is better than nothing and can remove some of the plaque on the surface of your teeth.

5. Bronze yourself a fuller bosom by smudging a dab of highlighter over the swell at the top of your bra.

6. Body brush every single morning before you take a shower. It will make you aware of your body as well as eliminate toxins.

7. To make your fragrance last, apply a body lotion first. It creates a foundation on which your scent can linger.

8. Uplift your day by dropping two drops of grapefruit and lemon essential oil into the bottom of your shower tray. The steam will lift the revitalising aromas for you to breathe in.

9. Posture is so much more important than make-up. Physical therapists encourage you to picture your head as a weightless balloon floating on top of your spine.

10. An instant big-date bust-toning tip: dip your bust in a cold water! Fill the sink with cold-as-you-dare water, then plunge. Blood will rush to the surface of the skin, giving a rosy glow and temporarily tightening the area.

11. Use a tongue scraper to keep your tongue clean. Remember, it's on show as much as your teeth.

12. Kick your shoes off as soon as you walk in the door. Shoes inhibit the form and function of the foot. And now your feet are nicely pedicured, you'll be proud to show them off.

13. Forgo acrylic nails. They stunt natural nail growth and make the nails weaker and more prone to splits.

14. If one nail breaks, cut them all down to the same length. Consistency is the key.

15. Soft and lightly polished nails will keep fresher looking for longer.

16. Use your foot buffer to buff any rough skin on elbows and knees.

17. If you are having a professional manicure, take along your own nail polish. This will make it easier for at-home touch-ups.

18. Keep your sense of smell open when travelling. Local fragrances can be irresistible and impossible to buy back home.

19. If your ankles are puffy, raise them higher than your head and drink a diuretic tea such as dandelion.

20. Enjoy wearing colours on your toes that you would never get away with on your fingertips.

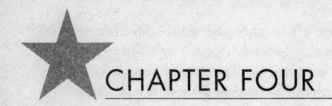

CHAPTER FOUR

How to get to hair heaven (and never come back)

'Hairstyle is the final tip-off whether or not a woman really knows herself.'
Hubert de Givenchy

Women and their hair: can there be any relationship more complex, intense and turbulent? In some ways our hair can be likened to a lover: one minute we can fall in lust with it, the next we hate it with a searing passion. We spend time talking about it, brushing it, stroking it, twirling it and becoming frustrated by it. Generally hair is the first thing we notice about a person, as it's there to attract the opposite sex – hair growth is even said to be stimulated by sexual activity, or just the expectation of it. When a woman wants to feel provocative she lets her hair down, when she wants to assert her independence she gets it cut or pulls it back. Great-looking hair is a way of flaunting your attractiveness and confidence.

And if your hair isn't the way you want it, you actually don't feel great. Years ago I interviewed a woman whose hair had suffered at the hands of a 'cowboy' hairdresser. He left her with chemical burns on her scalp and hair loss. The whole experience was so traumatic for her that her doctor prescribed tranquillisers and at one stage she had insufficient confidence to even leave her house. 'I changed from an outgoing woman into somebody whose self-belief was eaten away by the condition of my hair. I thought I looked hideous,' she said. Although this is an extreme story, it just goes to show how deeply psychological hair is.

Luckily, most of us don't require serious hair therapy, but a few of us should be talked out of the hair rut we seemed to have landed ourselves in. Think about what your hairstyle currently says about you. Does it say 'mumsy hair', 'housewife hair', 'get ahead hair' or 'sexy hair'? If you haven't given your hair so much as a second thought for years, it probably isn't giving a great impression. Perhaps 'I can't be bothered hair'?

Because our hairstyle gives us an identity, a lot of us hang onto a style we adopted when we felt good about ourselves or when we felt at our most successful. It's only natural not to want to let that feeling go, but if your hairstyle is now way out of date, maybe you should move on. Making over hair doesn't have to mean a radical change. It can be as subtle as a change of parting or adding a smattering of highlights. Whatever it takes, this chapter shows you how to get on the well-tressed list.

Understanding a bad hair day

The phrase 'having a bad hair day' has effortlessly slipped into our language, reflecting the fact that it is a very real and true phenomenon. In fact so real has it become that it's even been investigated by Yale University in America. Far from viewing a bad hair day (BHD) as a condition exclusively suffered by pathetic hair-centred nuts, the study uncovered important findings across three psychological measures: reduced self-esteem, increased social insecurity and a diminished sense of being worthwhile as a person. Fascinatingly, it reported that a BHD significantly lowered our expectations of ourselves. On a BHD we view ourselves as less smart, less capable, more embarrassed and less sociable. And you thought it was just you!

Studies have also revealed that bad hair days (BHDs) leave over 65 per cent of women feeling depressed and ugly. Further research highlights the fact that 45 per cent of women have actually cried over a BHD and one in six can't even leave the house when suffering from one. In fact, it's one of the top reasons for taking a sneaky sickie off from work!

TIME TO DITCH *Being unprepared for sudden BHDs.*

 CHANGE IT NOW *Carry an emergency hair kit. Include simple grips and a travel-size bottle of your key styling product.*

THE THREE CAUSES OF HAIR TRAUMA
1. Nutritional deficiencies, illness and stress

Eating a wide variety of food will ensure that the essential nutrients are delivered to all areas of the body, including the follicles from which the hair grows. Hair can often miss out, though, as the major organs take the lion's share. So if hair is looking more than lank, vitamin and mineral supplementation maybe required.

The importance of a balanced diet is dramatically shown when dieting. Within eight to ten days, the hair becomes lifeless, which is due to the sudden changes in the tissue in which it lives.

2. Shampoos

Shampoos can cause GHH (grievous hair harm). Often they are too harsh and picked without a thought to the specific hair type. Hair that is washed three times a week, for example, will be washed over 1,000 times in a year. If a silk shirt were washed that amount of times there would hardly be any fabric left. So you can understand why it's important to lather up with the right product to keep your hair supple and shiny.

3. Hormones

I know hormones are often blamed for everything, but the condition of our hair can be affected by our menstrual cycle. High oestrogen levels within the body make skin bloom and hair become thicker and glossier. This hormone is in abundance up to mid-cycle (ovulation), around 13 days before your period, when your body is potentially preparing for pregnancy. After ovulation and then three to seven days before your period starts, oestrogen levels plummet and the hormone progesterone becomes dominant. This is when you start feeling pre-menstrual: body fluids thicken, bloating can be experienced and waxy secretions of the skin are increased. This all adds up to the hair becoming oilier and limper during this time.

Troubleshooting BHDs

★ Good hair days start in the shower. Don't spend those extra ten minutes in bed – get up and shampoo your hair.

★ Don't use brushes and combs with broken teeth. They rip the hair cuticle and lead to split ends.

★ Buy a great hat.

HOW TO GET HAIR REHAB

Consumer insights into how we treat our crowning glory make for hair-raising reading. Research by Sunsilk haircare reveals that women feel guiltier about mistreating their hair than about lying to their partner. But this doesn't stop our toxic hair habits. The same study goes on to divulge that almost a third of women regularly straighten their hair with a heated appliance, more than half will not go out without the use of some kind of hair appliance or styling product, two in five blowdry their hair on the hottest setting and a handful let friends – not hairdressers – cut their hair.

Now, I could easily stand up and say, 'Hello, my name is Jacqui and I'm a hair abuser' – who couldn't? But I know that my confession will only be made half-heartedly, as I will resort to any abuse to get my hair just the way I want it.

Hair worry is just one more worry we just don't need, so prepare to repair your hair. The first step to hair rehab is admitting to your abuse. The second is modifying your behaviour.

Let's get started! What are your hair sins and what are the heavenly hair solutions?

Constant Use of Hot Appliances

Hair can all too easily be caught up in a catch-22 situation, as blowdryers and straightening irons can make your style as well as wreck the condition of your hair. But an onslaught of hot-headed abuse will generally suck all the life out of hair, leaving it brittle and straw-like.

Heavenly hair solution: Wait until your hair is at least three-quarters dry before you wage war with the dryer. That way even if you use your dryer on a hot setting, the hair will spend less time under the heat. If you use a flat iron, make sure it's a ceramic one, as these are

gentler than the metal versions, and prep step hair
with a heat product for thermal protection. And
keep the irons moving – don't stop or your hair will
burn.

Ignoring Split Ends

You don't think split ends are important? Look at
them under a microscope: the split just keeps on going
right from the end of the hair to the root. Each hair is
divided into two. The result? A feathery-looking
appearance, reduced shine and in some cases the hair
actually looks shorter.

Heavenly hair solution: No amount of product can repair
split ends. The only thing you can do is have them cut
off regularly and use conditioning treatments that
revitalise weakened hair.

Cutting Your Own Hair

Take note that even the professionals do not cut their
own hair. Stylists train for years in cutting techniques
and it's an absolute skill. A DIY haircut often results
in embarrassment, painful growing out, tears and in
extreme cases a wig! Those who are tempted by scissors will undoubtedly end up with an uneven haircut,
as weight will be taken out of all the wrong places. It
is then very hard for a stylist to rectify the problem
without cutting off a whole lot more.

Heavenly hair solution: Stick with a professional hairdresser.

Being Addicted to Hair Products

Overuse of products can be as bad as not using any at all – hair can be left greasy and gasping for life. Just that extra squirt of mousse or a little bit more wax can take your style from lush to limp in seconds.

Heavenly hair solution: Use styling and finishing products minimally – even one product can be enough to finish the style – and just use enough to moisten your palms. Give your hair a weekly detox too with reviving or clarifying shampoos that work hard to wash away styling residue.

Lazy Conditioning

Apparently under 10 per cent of us are happy with the condition of our hair and that's not surprising when most of us seem to be conditioner shy. All hair, especially coloured hair, craves hydration, and that comes from conditioner.

Also, when we do use it, we never leave it on for long enough. You wouldn't apply moisture to your skin then rinse it off straight away, would you?

Heavenly hair solution: Take time to massage conditioner in from mid-length downwards or, if you have time, clip up your hair and leave the conditioner on for 10 minutes. The heat from your scalp will open the cuticles, letting moisturiser from the conditioner reach the inner hair shaft.

Not Rinsing Thoroughly

No time to rinse? Shame on you!

Heavenly hair solution: If you rinse your hair for long enough, the difference can be amazing. Stay under the shower spray for at least two minutes. Use tepid water too. Very hot water increases the action of the sebaceous glands and makes hair oily.

Brushing Wet Hair

Wet hair is very different from dry hair. The elasticity is buoyant when wet and can stretch hair up to a third of its length. Therefore it's much, much weaker and more vulnerable to breakage.

Heavenly hair solution: To avoid this, take a wide-toothed comb and start combing from the ends of the hair upwards. This way tangles will gently be teased out rather than dragged down and damaged by a brush.

How to have a fabulous hair affair

'Some of the worst mistakes of my life have been haircuts.'
Jim Morrison

If there's one person every woman needs in her life it's a trusted hairstylist. This person has to be up to speed with your lifestyle and sensitive to your needs and emotions. One woman I know was told by a very insensitive stylist that she would never suit short hair as she was too flat-chested! A good stylist will also know how to read your mind and have the confidence to talk you out of ideas as well as encourage them.

One of the catalysts to having a drastic hair change is when a relationship has finished – call it a breakover. But only an astute stylist will know if a drastic hair change will be right at that time. One top hairdresser once told me a regular client suddenly hated her brunette hair and demanded he turn it platinum blonde. He was horrified. It was only after talking it through with her that he discovered her husband had run off with a blonde.

A similar story was also told to me by another hairdresser (I do so love these gossipy salon chats). A woman had asked for her waist-length hair to be cut short, short, short and the stylist had flatly refused, as she didn't have the fine facial features to pull this kind of look off. Upon using a little prying hair therapy, the stylist uncovered that the client was feeling insecure as her wayward partner had eyes for a woman with a very short crop. Funnily enough, upon her next visit, the 'other' woman plumped for hair extensions.

In situations like these, change your man, not your mane! But if you're in a hair rut, a change might be just what you need.

★ **TIME TO DITCH** *Scraping hair back with an elastic band. The band will cut into the hair, cause tension and lead to breakage and even hair loss.*

★ **CHANGE IT NOW** *Use a fabric-covered band. They're kinder and chicer. Or, for instant glamour, sleek hair into a ponytail then take a section of the hair, wrap it around the base of your ponytail and pin it.*

According to a lot of stylists, the reason why many women get stuck in a hair rut is purely because they're frightened of losing their length – the Rapunzel syndrome. If that's the case, be gutsy and prepare yourself for something stronger – that's what making over your hair is all about. But don't panic – dropping five years in the time it takes to cut your hair can be as simple as adding a few layers or cutting in a fringe.

THINGS TO TELL YOUR STYLIST BEFORE THE SCISSORS

The golden rule for fabulous hair is never to let the hairstyle wear you. You'll feel out of control with your look. When you go into the salon, wise up to the idea that you're actually buying a haircut. It's just like buying a skirt or shirt. Like these, a haircut has to do more than just look nice on the first try-on, it has to fit into your everyday life as well. The secret is telling your stylist about the life you lead.

 TIME TO DITCH *Talking inches with your hairdresser!*

 CHANGE IT NOW *'An inch from the length' may vary a great deal. It's best to show your stylist how short you want to go.*

HANDLING YOUR STYLIST

★ To find a stylist, go by word of mouth or choose the best-looking and best-staffed salon in your area. Someone who has invested in their business will be offering good haircuts.

★ Say how much time and money you're willing to spend on your hair.

★ Tell them your profession. A good stylist will give less edgy cuts to someone who banks than someone who works in a trendy shop.

★ Reveal past cuts you've hated or loved. Show and tell with photographs.

★ Be appointment aware. Avoid booking your stylist first

thing in the morning (hangovers) or last thing in the evening (tired). Mid-morning to late afternoon will see your stylist at their freshest and most creative.

★ Play the word game. Pick three words that describe the cut you want.

★ Don't focus too much on chit-chat on a first cut. You want to be aware of the style you're getting, not discussing where you're going on holiday.

★ Look and learn. Pay attention to how your stylist styles your hair. Ask which products they're using. A good stylist will never get bored of answering your questions.

★ Be yourself. This is not an appointment to dress up or down. Stick to your style and never wear a polo neck for an appointment.

A Heavenly Client Will Be:

★   Realistic about their hair

★   Able to explain what they want

★   On time

★   Viewing the stylist as a friend, not an enemy

★   At all costs avoiding the words: 'I'd rather visit the dentist than go to the hairdresser's!'

The six classic styles

n my experience there are six great haircuts that crop up over and over again – a bit like *Groundhog Day* for hair. One of them is bound to suit you. Here they are, in no particular order:

LONG WITH A FRINGE

This is a way you can keep your length and still makeover your style. Fringes can give a dramatic new spin. Hairdressers say that they can change someone's look totally. A fringe will always make a woman look younger and is a great way of softening features. Plus it's a way of keeping hair long without swamping the face with hair, and there really is a fringe type for everyone, regardless of face shape.

Forget Botox, Wear a Fringe

★ If you have a long face, a blunt fringe can make it look smaller, as well as make a strong statement.
★ For an oval or small face, try a wispy fringe that hits just above the eyes.
★ For every other face shape, go for a long and layered fringe. You can play around with it by sweeping or clipping it to the side.

A Quick Lesson on Trimming your own Fringe

Okay, okay, I know I said, 'Never ever cut your own hair,' but there are always exceptions to the rules. As long as you initially get your fringe cut in professionally you can afford to trim it up in between salon visits. How do you do it?

★ Wash your hair.

★ Section off a one-inch thick section (that is, the length of one eyebrow). (Never cut the fringe wider than your eyebrows – it looks scary.)

★ Sit in natural daylight in front of a mirror.

★ Comb the section flat.

★ Do not look up at what you are doing, look straight ahead in the mirror. If you look up, the raising of your eyebrows will take the fringe up far too short.

★ Cut the fringe to one inch longer than the length you want it to be dry. This will allow for the natural fall of the hair when it's not wet.

★ Do not use kitchen, garden or nail scissors. Buy scissors for cutting hair.

THE BOB

This is an all-time classic that first made its style debut in the 1920s. Think Louise Brooks. The original bob was worn straight and flat on top or with a Marcel wave, but since then this style has been invented many times over, with Vidal Sassoon making it his own with striking asymmetrical lines.

If your image cries out for a chic overhaul, then this is the style for you. It's ideal for an oval or heart-shaped face and instantly draws attention to the cheeks and eyes. It can look very flattering. A graduated cut, so the front sections are longer than the back, will keep it looking modern. For a younger look, try a swingy cut where the hair is slightly sliced into. That will also give a softer feel.

THE PIXIE CUT

For some people, the shorter the hair, the hotter the look. It takes guts to go from long to short, but results can be fabulous. A short cut needn't look aggressive either – a clever and sensitive cut can make it very feminine. It's all in your attitude, bone structure and face shape.

Let me be frank: short hair can look a disaster on someone with a long face, a prominent nose or big ears. A round face can be a problem too. Too short and it can look positively moon-like.

Ultimately, a pixie cut or crop suits those with fine and delicate features – think Mia Farrow, Twiggy and Jean Seberg in their heyday (or should it be 'hair day'?) – and it always looks best a little ruffled, otherwise it can look too severe and helmet-like. Waxes are great to create definition, but the hair should never looked puffed and fluffed.

Going short can be liberating, but if you're unsure, take it in stages. That way you can adjust to a shorter length gradually. And remember: short hair is ultimately more work than long. It's less versatile and you just can't scoop it up into a bun when you haven't time to style it. Ask yourself, 'Can I handle it?'

LAYERED AND LONG

If you want to vary your style, learn to love layers. They are a great way to bring body and swing to hair without doing anything too drastic. The key is for your stylist to create them in proportion to your current length and texture. Most stylists look upon layering as the most versatile styling tool they have, as it can totally change the look of a style. One-length hair is very limiting, not to mention a little boring, but by adding layers you can actually make the style look longer.

To give shoulder-length hair a sexy I've-been-rolling-about-in-bed vibe, layers can begin at the cheekbones, or on longer hair they can even start as low as the chin.

When blowdrying, work with your natural texture and accentuate the chipping in of the layers with a small drop of gloss serum run through the length with your fingers.

THE SHAG

Once you've got over asking your stylist for a shag, bear in mind it's been dubbed 'the haircut that flatters everyone' and has been worn on the most fashionable of heads from Goldie Hawn to Meg Ryan to Jennifer Aniston.

Shags are essentially well-engineered messes with lots of seemingly haphazard layers and very pronounced pieces on the ends and sides. The scoop on this sexy low-maintenance style is it can be worn long or short, as long as it's kept choppy. And it's an especially great cut if you have a wide jawline or face. The choppiness of it will make it look slimmer.

Another advantage of this style is it's so easy to maintain.

If you're in a rush you can practically wash it, rough dry it, texturise it with a small amount of wax or pomade and go, go, go.

CONTROLLED CURLS

The way to make curls look modern is a clever cut to help maximise curl formation. And for this it's back to layers, as they eliminate weight and lift curls. Curly hair that's kept all one length can look very unruly and bushy.

When styling, curls need to be cultivated with a taming cream, so look for the keys words 'curl control', and when drying a diffuser is not an option, it's essential to help define the curls. Tip your head forwards and dry underneath first. The less fiddling you do with the hair the better; just let it sit in the diffuser cup. Don't ruffle it with your hands, as this encourages frizz. And never brush your curls – just use your fingers to gently break them apart.

Because curly hair has a curved surface, it's hard for it to reflect light. Overcome this problem by running a little serum through from the mid-length to the end of the hair.

Cut to the Quick

★ A blunt cut is best suited to fine hair. It will give the illusion that it's thicker.

★ Layers and graduation suit medium-textured hair because they add softness.

★ Thick hair needs the weight taken out with layers to stop it from hanging too heavy.

> ★ Wavy hair needs a cut to maximise natural movement, not one that works against it.
> ★ Light layers encourage great curl formation with curly hair.

Making a colour statement

If you want a head of hair that stands out in a crowd, then look to colour. I think even the most expensive cut is incomplete without an injection of colour to enhance depth, texture and shine.

Colour is hot and you'd better believe it when I reveal that three-quarters of women use hair colour as a way to boost their confidence, both in their working and personal lives. A leading psychologist has even gone as far as to say that hair colour is one of the strongest communicators we have.

A survey by Clairol confirms this. They asked the question: 'Does hair colour play a role in how women are viewed in their personal and professional lives?' And the answer was a resounding *yes*. Their 'Colourwonderful' survey revealed that brunettes are seen as leaders and are perceived as trustworthy, practical and self-confident. However, they are also seen as more argumentative, less likely to take risks and less glamorous than other hair colours. Although all is not lost: the survey revealed that if the CEO of a company could hire only one woman based on her hair colour it would be a brunette.

As for blondes, not surprisingly they were seen as the

most glamorous and most likely to be noticed by the opposite sex. They were also observed to be the wealthiest and the colour that most enjoyed being pampered.

But despite the attention blondes attract, men believe redheads have better love lives than blondes or brunettes. Just over half of all women, given the choice, would become red for a day.

Although the results of this survey make for entertaining reading, they also illustrate how hair colour speaks volumes in terms of how we are viewed by others. So, whether you want to max out your natural hair colour or change it completely, how can you use these colour stereotypes to your best advantage?

 TIME TO DITCH *Fruit or vegetables (aubergine or damson for instance) when talking colour.*

 CHANGE IT NOW *Think animal (mink) or food (chocolate or caramel). That makes for a warmer and more seductive colour thought.*

Big on Blonde

People often say that being blonde is a state of mind rather than a hair colour, and I would agree. Personally, when I'm blonde I feel more outgoing, but when I'm darker I feel a little more subdued. I miss my blonde hair pretty quickly and after a few weeks always go back to my colourist so he can pump up the colour a little.

If blonde is your thing, move away from the ash, beige and sandy shades that can look flat and go more for the gorgeous honeys, caramels and toffee-cream hues which can either by applied as 'slices' through the hair to define the haircut or just around the hairline to give a curtain effect of blonde framing the face. These colours and techniques especially heat up cool skin tones and bring out the colour in blue and green eyes.

If you decide to reach for the bleach and have an all-over colour, be prepared to strike up an intimate relationship with your colourist every four to six weeks for root retouches.

Bring on the Brunettes

With so much talk about blondes being more fun and oozing sex appeal, you would think brunettes never turn heads. Don't you believe it: brunettes can look stunning.

Although brunette hair reflects the light and makes for a shiny, rich block of colour, it can be a hue that looks a little too dense and solid. A touch of colour can really enhance it by delivering a sense of lightness and movement for a three-dimensional hair experience.

The general rule is to only go two to three shades lighter or darker than your natural hair colour, and I think this is very true for brunettes. Go too dark and it knocks all colour from your complexion and go too light and it can look at odds with your skin tone, especially if you're olive-skinned.

Warm bronze and chestnut tones can look fabulous when woven through the hair and can enhance brown and hazel eyes as well as add warmth to neutral skin tones. Strawberry or golden streaks can look good on brunettes who want to inject a touch of blonde, especially when placed around the hairline.

In between colour visits a colour gloss can be used to amplify colour and give hair shine.

Revving Up for Red

'Traffic stopping' can be the only way to describe a great-looking redhead. Plus red is such a versatile colour. Whatever your natural base shade, adding hints of golden copper and vibrant tones of auburn will be more than possible.

A rich copper red will instantly lift green and hazel eyes and complement a pinky skin tone. But the beauty of red has to be in its strength, so if you're natural, don't be afraid to play it up.

There are almost no fashion rules when it comes to red and there's no feeling better than pulling off a vibrant red with slices of blonde tones scattered through. Just be aware that red colour molecules are released more quickly during shampooing. A good tip for longer-lasting colour is to rinse hair with cool water, as this will not dilute the colour molecules so fast.

Shades of Grey

Admit it, when you first discovered a grey hair, you probably felt you were getting old. Grey hair is associated with ageing, which is why there's such a booming trade in home hair colorants. Eighty per cent of women who dye their hair do so to hide the grey. So, what should you do to cover it up?

If your hair is only 15–20 per cent grey, then a semi-permanent is fine, or if it's a subtle disguise you want, look to high or lowlights that help blend the offending grey hairs in with your natural colour. However, if your hair is a higher percentage of grey then the only effective way of covering it is to use a permanent colour.

 TIME TO DITCH *Being locked into the hair colour of your youth.*

 CHANGE IT NOW *Your skin pigment changes over the years, so check out what your skin and hair are doing now. And then bring them both together.*

SHOULD YOU DYE AT HOME?

Although the hair dyes you find sitting on the shelves today are far more sophisticated than those of just a few years back, colouring is a skill and should be treated as such. There's nothing worse than ending up with 'supermarket' hair. By that I mean you've pulled a permanent dye off the shelf and look like you've literally poured it over your head. It's way too bright or too dark, looks completely solid (professional colourists can use up to three colours on your hair) and does nothing for your complexion.

I understand there are several advantages to home colouring, one of them being cost and the other being that you can colour your hair when it suits you without having to sit for hours in the salon. But sometimes it's better to be a slave to the salon than a slave to a look you have to wait to grow out. If you do choose to go it alone, though, here are some tips:

How to Avoid Scary Home Colour

★ Read the instructions twice. This will ensure that you know exactly how to apply the colour and whether it's right for your hair.

★ Dress for the occasion. Put on an old shirt and drape a towel over your shoulders.

★ Always, always do a strand test.

★ Always colour on clean dry hair. Styling residue can affect the colour.

★ Don't expect the colour to cover grey unless it says so.

★ Never by guided by the model on the box. Use the chart on the back as a guide to what shade you can realistically expect to end up with.

★ Always wear the gloves provided.

★ Apply Vaseline around your hairline and the tips of your ears to block staining.

★ Never apply colour to damaged or overprocessed hair such as permed or heavily bleached hair. The hair will be very porous and the colour will soak in, leaving you with a very different result from what you expected.

★ In the event of a colour mishap, wash your hair immediately with a clarifying shampoo, as this will help remove excess colour. Call the hotline on the back of the box before doing anything else to your hair.

★ Highlighting kits can spell trouble. It takes years to perfect the art of highlighting and it's certainly not something that can be achieved in an afternoon.

GET GORGEOUS: 20 INSTANT MAKEOVER HAIR TIPS

1. Touch, tease and twiddle your hair as little as possible after styling it. It will lose its shape and quickly become greasy.

2. The best way to save time styling short layered hair is to look in the mirror and see how it's behaving. Layers can be manipulated easily, but a good eye is needed. Dip fingertips into wax and work with your natural texture to style.

3. When using a hairdryer, switch to the cool button just before finishing. Apply too much heat and your scalp will perspire, causing your hair to lose its bounce.

4. Hair masks are excellent for stressed-out hair and reward it with oodles of glossy shine and a better-behaved texture.

5. Flip your parting and change it to the opposite side. Not only will it give your hair an instant makeover, but it will also give it more volume.

6. Refresh hair instantly and eliminate smoke and cooking smells by spritzing your favourite fragrance on a hairbrush and brushing it through.

7. Give short hair a midday revival by misting it with water and working a little product through from roots to ends.

8. Starched and lacquered hair makes you look dated. Loosen it up to drop the years.

9. If you have parched hair, swap your cotton pillowcase for a satin one. It will soak up fewer of the hair's natural oils.

10. Splurge on good professional shampoos. Using poor-quality products is like washing your hair with soap or washing-up liquid. Use colour-boosting shampoos for coloured hair. Colour fades when you wash it and these shampoos help put the pigments back.

11. For a sexy style for shoulder-length hair, dry it only at the roots and along the hairline for volume and let the rest air dry. When it is dry, treat it with a serum or a styling crème for polish.

12. Putting a great pair of sunglasses on top of your head is the modern equivalent of the Alice band. Sunglasses can be one of the chicest hair accessories.

13. Sex up long hair and become a pin-up girl: show off your neck by scooping and pinning your hair up into a mussed-up bun and pulling out random sections.

14. A black-tie do doesn't have to equal big hair. Overstyled hair looks as if you're trying too hard. Rough it up a little so it doesn't look too well-bred.

15. Pick the right conditioner for your hair. The thicker your hair, the creamier you want your conditioner to be. The finer it is, the lighter you want it.

16. Don't go overboard with hair straighteners. When it's too straight your hair can take on a Barbie doll acrylic look. Use hair irons to flip the ends up a little.

17. The conditions inside aeroplanes are incredibly drying, so post-flight lather up with a moisturising shampoo to renourish the hair.

18. Clip-in hair extensions make for a great one-night hair stand.

19. Never rely on sunshine or lemon juice to give your hair highlights unless you want an uneven bleached and dried-out mess. Get sun-kissed highlights before you go on holiday.

20. If you find you have to wear more make-up to make your hair colour work with your skin, it's the wrong hue for you.

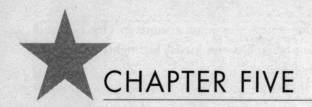

CHAPTER FIVE

Making over your nutrition

'Never eat more than you can lift.'
Miss Piggy

Food should be one of life's great pleasures, along with a round of cocktails with your girlfriends. But too often it is caught up in a web of remorse and self-loathing. We are all too willing to be seduced by pictures of svelte celebrities. We get wrapped up in what we should look like instead of who we are and this can fast-breed body insecurity. And then there's the dress size fascism to deal with. Who hasn't at some point felt a social outcast when forced to ask a shop assistant to dig out a size 14 or 16 from the storeroom when the shop only hangs out 8s or 10s?

In a quest to obtain the perfect figure, the average woman is unrealistic about how much weight she needs to lose, influenced in part by icons who like to while away their time being slaves to freaky diets. A supermodel typically has a body mass index (BMI) – that's weight divided by height – of less than 20 per cent. That is medically classed as being underweight. An acceptable weight range is actually up to 25. That allows a woman of 5ft 6in to weigh in at anything between 8st 8lb and 10st 10lb.

Working Out your BMI

★ Convert your weight to kilograms by dividing your weight in pounds by 2.2.

★ Convert your height (in inches only) to metres by dividing it by 39.4, then square the answer.

★ Divide answer one by answer two. This is your BMI.

★ For instance, if your weight is 65 kilograms and height 1.68 metres, first multiply 1.68 by 1.68. That comes to 2.82. Next divide 65 by your answer (2.82). Your BMI is 23.0.

More and more we are being shown anatomical impossibilities as the ideal, and ultimately these can be very stressful and damaging to live up to. Which is why we all should be striving for a 'happy' weight instead.

A happy weight is one where you feel comfortable in your own skin, you eat healthily, exercise regularly and can move freely and easily without breathlessness. It's also about having a realistic understanding of your body's make-up. In reality, there is very little you can do to outwit your genes. If you're predisposed to having 'big bones', you're never going to wind up as a designer's clotheshorse. Once you stop beating yourself up about reaching an improbable weight for you and bring mind and body together, you'll be well on your way to becoming a happy weight and a happier person.

But apart from beating body envy, we have to remember that nutrition, especially when made over into power nutrition, can fight illness, prevent ageing and help your body not only perform but also look its best.

Everyone knows that shedding pounds is only half the battle. The secret is maintaining your happy weight long term. When it comes to eating, most people are driven by what they see, not by how they feel, so without getting all touchy feely about it, this chapter looks at the relationship you have with food and how you can improve on it.

My personal motto? Eat healthily and be happy.

Making over your weight-loss plan

The first lesson to address is the reason *why* you want to lose weight in the first place. If it's because you've gradually piled on the weight and now can't fit into your favourite pair of jeans, then good on you. Shed it and feel fabulous. If it's because you think that once you've fought the flab you'll be smarter, more popular and will get promoted, then you're at greater risk of piling it back on again.

Psychologists reveal that it's common for overweight people to put their lives on hold. They tell themselves that when the unwanted weight is lost, their lives will change. But when their lives don't change, they become disheartened and give up.

We've all heard those motivational tales of a woman who went on a diet and lost 10 stone in 10 months, but how much did she manage to keep off 10 years down the line?

Experts say if you're serious about dropping a dress size or two, then be prepared for problems before they surface. You'll be more successful at long-term weight loss if you map out your goals before you start counting the calories. Think of it as handling a business proposal – you set goals, develop a strategy and then take steps to put it into action.

FIND YOUR INCENTIVE

Ask yourself: 'How will I benefit from losing weight?' If you can't answer this question, your diet will certainly fail. Trying to lose weight with no clear incentive is a waste of time.

Once you have an incentive, it will determine your approach. For instance, if your goal is to drop half a stone, then maybe dropping the dessert is all that's necessary. Losing a couple of stone because you want to lower your risks of ill health requires bigger changes and maybe the enlisting of a slimming club to address your daily eating habits.

BE PATIENT

It took time to gain weight, so don't expect to drop it in minutes. Many people spend years trying to slim because they don't have the patience to stick to a healthy-eating plan long term.

If losing weight sensibly means losing a pound or two a week, calculate when you can expect to reach your goal. Write it down in your diary. It's probably a lot further away than you thought. But if you try and lose weight through quick-fix diets you're more likely to fail in the long run.

BE REALISTIC

Okay, you may have been lighter five years ago, but remind yourself that women naturally put on weight with age. Or, if you want to reach a weight you slimmed down to for a special occasion, remember how hard you had to work for it.

You also have to ask, 'What is going on in my life?' People often conjure up a lot of reasons why they can't lose weight and usually they're simple excuses. But sometimes major life changes like having a baby, divorcing or moving, for example, make it hard to rethink your eating habits. You may not always be ready to take on the challenge of successful weight loss.

BE HONEST ABOUT YOUR CALORIE NEEDS

Figure out how many calories you consume on an average day. Write down everything – and I mean *everything* – you ate in the past 24 hours. And don't forget drinks, snacks and bits of food stolen from other people's plates.

Now buy yourself a calorie counter book and roughly add up your intake on just one day. A woman's daily calorie allowance is 2,000 a day. How much over your daily limit are you?

Here's the lowdown on the fat gain: for each extra 3,500 calories above your daily limit you will put on 1lb of fat. If you overeat just 500 calories a day for a week – for instance that could be a Danish pastry at 287 calories and a Mars bar at 294 calories – you will gain 1lb of fat. If you overeat by 1,000 calories a day for one week, that's an extra 2lbs of fat you will be wearing if there's no change in your activity level to work off all those extra pleasures.

WORK OUT A SENSIBLE EATING PLAN

Diets can be likened to relationships – you should keep trying until you find 'the one'. Not all eating regimes fit all. Look at the lifestyle that you lead along with your foodie likes and dislikes. A plan that requires a home-cooked lunch won't work for someone that works in an office with only a microwave for company and someone who craves pasta won't be happy with a high-protein diet. This is asking for failure before you've even begun.

WEIGH YOURSELF LESS

Your weight varies from day to day, so you'll be disheartened if you don't see the scales dropping. Plus, if you're exercising, remember that muscle weighs more than fat. Personally, I chucked out the scales years ago and measure my happy weight by the tightness of my waistbands.

DON'T VIEW LAPSES AS DEFEATS

Everyone falls off their eating plan at some point. So what? Just get back on it the next day or the next week. Don't be hard on yourself. Worrying about your weight can make you fatter because it makes you miserable and therefore more likely to reach for comfort food. Worrying about a problem makes you less able to solve it.

 TIME TO DITCH *Personal body bashing. It's unconstructive and leads to low self-esteem.*

CHANGE IT NOW *Talk yourself up. Remind yourself you have an amazing body and really look after it instead of filling it with junk.*

Bust your biggest diet blunders

OUTSMART YOUR CRAVINGS

Science may debate whether cravings are biological or psychological, but one thing's for sure: they are hard to break and can ruin any weight-loss plan you're embarking upon.

First, don't ignore a craving, it will only make it stronger. And finally find a right time to tackle it. Do it when life is looking up (you'll be stronger), rather than when you're feeling down.

Here are some common cravings and how to beat them:

Caffeine

Addiction: We crave caffeine when we're bored or stressed. It heightens alertness but in the long term can result in fatigue and nervousness.

Blasting your crave: Caffeine is hidden in numerous things, including cold remedies and fizzy drink. But tackling your coffee fix is a start. Reduce your intake by one cup every fourth day.

Carbohydrates

Addiction: Refined carbs such as those found in bread and pastries hook you in by triggering a fast release of feel-good brain chemicals.

Blasting your crave: Eat small meals containing some protein every few hours to keep blood sugar levels steady. Skipping meals can cause levels to drop, leaving you craving processed carbohydrates.

Chocolate

Addiction: Apart from the fact it gives an instant sugar high, chocolate can be a hard addiction to break as it has a lot of amazing chemicals that mimic the feelings brought on during sex and happiness.

Blasting your crave: There are two solutions. Eat a few squares of dark, organic chocolate rich in cocoa solids. It's so strong your crave will be met by eating less. And the second? Have sex!

DIET BLUNDERS

'My doctor told me to stop having intimate dinners for four. Unless there are three other people.'

Orson Welles

I don't really like the word 'diet', as it instantly spells out deprivation to me. You only have to tell yourself you're on a diet and instantly a conveyor belt of things you can't have goes through your mind. The majority of us would be more than happy with our bodies if we could just shift a few pounds and this can be done without necessarily taking huge food groups out of your diet or banning every substance that excites the eye or tastebuds. The trick is to overcome common diet saboteurs.

BIG PORTIONS

This is the biggie (excuse the pun). Many experts are concerned that uncontrolled portions are contributing to an obesity epidemic. It's a practice that's been dubbed 'portion distortion' – typical servings of food have increased in size by up to seven times in 20 years.

So many foods today are super-sized that we're seduced by quantity rather than quality and along the way forget about the calorie content. Take a chocolate bar. We could get the taste sensation from a standard size, but go for king size and you effortlessly add 150 calories.

And while mega portions at restaurants have become a familiar part of food marketing, they have also crept into home cooking. We quickly get used to large portions when eating out and want more when cooking at home to keep us satisfied.

How to Downsize Your Portions

★ Limit the amount of food you put out for a meal. If a recipe serves six and only three will be eating, remove the extra portions and freeze them for later.

★ Health professionals teach people to visually

balance their food on their plate by composing their meals of 1/3 or more fruit and vegetables, 1/3 or more wholegrains and potatoes, about 2/15 animal protein or alternatives, 1/15 fatty food and sugar and 2/15 milk and dairy.

★ Eat slowly. It takes about 20 minutes for the signal indicating that you're full to go from your stomach to your brain.

★ Once you've finished eating, clear the table. Seconds never taste as good and bump up your portion size.

★ Avoid buffets. It's much harder to practise portion control when it's an all-you-can-eat.

★ Take a diet lesson from the French. Petite isn't just a dress size, it's their portion size too. Their obesity rate is much lower than those of the US and UK.

DRINKING LOTS OF CALORIES

Why is it we never think of drinks as calories, just refreshing liquid? While modifying your diet is half the battle, remember that more calories can lurk in the wet stuff.

A typical day can roughly go something like this: caffe latte early morning (132 calories), large glass of orange juice with lunch (99 calories), two cups of sweet tea early afternoon (40 calories each) and a can of Coke late afternoon (129 calories) and two glasses of wine in the evening (75 calories each). Grand total: 590 calories.

So how can your liquid intake be improved on? Well, take a little less orange juice and you could reduce your intake to 66 calories, use skimmed milk in your latte and you'll drop another 66 calories. Take only one spoonful of sugar in your tea and save another 40 calories. Choose Diet Coke over regular and save another 128 calories. And limit yourself to one glass of wine. Or the alternative? Drink water. It's only motive is to keep you hydrated and it is calorie free.

BINGEING

We all do it. We're home late, exhausted from the day and drawn to the biscuit tin before we even start cooking our main meal.

When thinking about eating, ask yourself how hungry you actually are. Just one biscuit, for instance, will usually stop the hunger pangs before you sit down and eat. If you eat when you aren't hungry, your body will store that food as fat.

Weekend bingeing is a common pitfall too. People tend to go overboard on alcohol, snack foods and desserts over those two days. A little treat certainly won't hurt, but tucking away an extra 500 calories or more on Saturday and Sunday could hamper the good eating habits you've adopted in the week. Make choices: a glass of wine with dinner or a dessert, but not both.

 TIME TO DITCH *Eating by candlelight.*

 CHANGE IT NOW *Turn up the lights. Putting your food in the spotlight can help fight the urge to overeat.*

SUPERMARKET CRUISING WHEN FAMISHED

Try not to go shopping between 3 p.m. and 7 p.m. – the lull of the day when your blood sugar level is at its lowest. You'll only be tempted to buy on-the-go snacks.

Plan your meals for the next week. List the ingredients and try not to stray from them.

And beware: the bright sugary foods and alcohol are normally in the last aisle you come to. It's tempting to load up when fatigued and buy anything just so you can go home. But there's nothing to stop you starting at the far end of the shop and working back to the healthier produce of fruit and vegetables.

PARTYING

I don't want to be a killjoy here, but party snacks such as peanuts and crisps distort your appetite regulation (especially when eaten along with alcohol), making you think you want to go on eating long after you're full. After a time, you just don't know whether you're hungry or not, so you just assume you are and nibble away your daily calorie allowance just from one bowl.

Before you go out, resolve to eat a small healthy meal such as an omelette, then keep away from the food table and hopefully your willpower will win through.

EATING WHAT YOU LIKE BECAUSE YOU WORK OUT

There's no doubt that working out is good for you, but it doesn't give you an open licence to pig out. Bear in mind that swimming, for instance, burns up around 175 calories

in half an hour and just one chocolate mini roll is 117 calories and eaten in one minute or less!

BEING LOVED UP
Although it's official that marriage makes you healthier,
unfortunately it also makes you fatter. A study published in
Social Science and Medicine in America found that women
who are newly married gain more weight than women who
stay single or have been married for some time.

For starters, calorie requirements differ widely between
men and women. Whereas men usually need 2,300–2,700
calories a day, women require only 1,600–2,400 a day. This
single factor accounts for many of the weight problems that
plague women. The pitfall that they commonly encounter
is competitive eating.

SKIPPING BREAKFAST
You may think ignoring breakfast may well save on calories,
but in fact those people who go to work on an empty
stomach generally have a higher fat intake than those who
sit down and breakfast like a king. The reason? If you skip
breakfast, mid-morning blood sugar levels will crash and
you're more likely to cave in and eat something sweet and
comforting like a Danish pastry. A good breakfast – wholemeal cereal, toast, yoghurt or fresh fruit – will supply you
with essential fibre and vitamins rather than refined carbohydrates and fat later in the morning.

TIME TO DITCH *Thinking of yourself as fat.*

 CHANGE IT NOW *Think of yourself as slim(mer) and you will start to believe it. Imagine yourself a dress size smaller and start moving like it. Keep that thought.*

Become a smart supermarket shopper

Warning: Supermarket shopping may be sabotaging your health without you even realising it.

'Supermarket seduction' I call it. And the marketing men have got it down to a fine art. It starts the minute you walk into the supermarket and the smell of fresh bread hits your nostrils as it is pumped through the air conditioning. Here's how to avoid being seduced and to shop smart.

THE PRODUCE AISLE

'Colourise' your meals: If you select at least one fruit or vegetable from each colour, you'll have most of your disease-fighting nutritional bases covered. That's because many of the plant compounds that protect against disease are primarily responsible for giving certain foods their vibrant hues. Dark green vegetables such as spinach or broccoli are loaded with nutrients such as vitamin A and C, for example, while red produce such as tomatoes and pink grapefruit contain lycopene, which guards against heart disease and some forms of cancer. Beta-carotene, another strong anti-cancer fighter, is found in orange fruit and vegetables such as peppers and tomatoes. If your diet is mostly beige – think potatoes and pasta – it will contain very little of these nutrients.

For vegetables, don't be put off by the frozen section. Frozen veg are the next best thing to fresh, as many are frozen right at the field within hours of being picked, guaranteeing more locked-in goodness than supposedly 'market fresh' produce.

Look for produce in season: Produce out of season will be imported and will have been harvested before being fully ripe in order to withstand being transported. By the time it actually lands on the supermarket shelf its nutrients will be depleted. Even better, for real freshness shop at farmers' markets, which are becoming ever more popular.

THE DAIRY AISLE

Swap full fat for reduced fat: What's cereal without milk? But instead of going for the full-fat kind, go for skimmed, which has half the calories. Be aware that most of the calories from cream will come from fat, two thirds of which is saturated and a major factor in heart disease.

Yoghurts are a good source of calcium but contain a lot of fat, much of which is saturated. Fruit yoghurts tend to contain a lot of sugar too, so avoid if possible or limit your intake. To get your calcium fix, go for low-fat yoghurts.

Think about your cheeses: Cheese is deemed a protein food, but weight for weight many cheeses contain more fat than protein. Even half-fat cheeses may contain up to half of their calories as fat. If you are a cheese lover, then go for cheeses such as Stilton. Although still calorific, the taste is so strong you only need a little piece to get your fix.

Stock up on eggs: A small egg is only 69 calories and protein friendly. Although eggs are high in cholesterol, food experts say this should not present a problem for anyone whose blood cholesterol level is normal. So eggs make for a quick nutritious snack.

Dress salads carefully: Pouring dressing all over your salad is the quickest way to sabotage your efforts at eating healthily. Just two tablespoons of Thousand Island dressing adds up to 194 calories and 20 grams of fat. Drench your salad in it and see your supposedly low-cal green salad topping the calorie count of a platter of nachos! Blue cheese dressing is even worse: two tablespoons drizzled over greens and you're swallowing 228 calories and 23 grams of fat.

For a healthier option it's back to the produce aisle. Lemon and lime juices squeezed over salads are a great low-fat option. When buying bottled, take a minute to read the label. Find the low-fat, low-calorie alternative to your favourite dressing.

THE BAKERY AISLE

Choose a healthy loaf: The key word here is 'wholegrain' or 'wholemeal'. Wholegrain bread delivers a rich, nuttier taste while adding a dose of fibre to your diet. And don't be misled by the description of 'hearty' or 'multigrain'. Bread made with wholegrains lists wholewheat flour first on the ingredients list. For additional nutritional benefits, look for wholegrain breads with added nuts and seeds.

White bread is naturally much lower in vitamins and minerals than wholemeal bread.

Pass on the muffins: Avoid giant muffins and scones. Just one has several servings' worth of fat and calories.

THE MEAT COUNTER

Play the word game: When choosing cuts of meat, choose anything that has 'loin' in the name, as it will be the leanest cut. That's cuts like tenderloin, sirloin or loin chops.

Buy with skin: You may be tempted to buy poultry cuts without the skin to save on fat and calories, but the skin keeps the meat moist by packing in natural juices while cooking. Just remove it afterwards. And be aware that dark meat cut from the thigh and legs sections is higher in fat than white meat from the breast.

Pick fresh-looking meat: Meat should never look off-colour (grey), but be dark red or pale pink. It's often smart to pay a little more for organic meat (at least you know it was slaughtered healthy and 'happy') for better quality.

Look for reduced-fat hams: Believe it or not, these often taste just as good as full-fat meat, especially when eaten with coarse-grain mustard. The type of preparation – roasting, baking or smoking – has little effect on the calorie and fat content unless sweet glazes such as honey syrup have been used.

THE FISH COUNTER

Keep it plain: Low-fat, low-calorie fish includes plain-cooked white fish such as cod, haddock and brill. These are also a good source of protein, vitamins and minerals and are ideal for those trying to slim. Oily fish such as herring, mackerel, sardines and salmon are some of the few nutritional sources of the omega-3 polyunsaturated fatty acids that help to prevent heart disease. Mix in a little oily fish with the low-fat fish up to three times a week for a well-balanced diet.

The leaner guide to dining out

'I never worry about diets. The only carrots that interest me are the number you get in a diamond.'
Mae West

Finding well-balanced and healthy food that is good to eat takes planning at the supermarket, but at the restaurant table it can be a minefield. Leaving your meal to a chef means you never quite know what's in your food. It doesn't land on your table with a list of ingredients and a detailed calorie and fat content.

According to a university study, people who eat out more than three times a week consume nearly a third more calories a day than those who eat in restaurants once a week or less.

If you're planning a meal out, or even a takeaway, and you're looking at your waistline, then it pays to become an undercover menu sleuth. Here's the lowdown on some of the most popular dine-outs.

INDIAN

Take the favourite: Chicken korma, pilau rice and naan give a grand total of 1,315 calories with 70 grams of fat. That's a woman's fat allowance for the whole day gone in one meal. It's the creamy sauce and extra fat in the rice and bread that bump up the calories. The secret is to opt for dry curries which are low in fat, such as tandooris that are marinated in yoghurt, not cream, along with a side order of plain boiled rice. Alternatively, go for dhal dishes that boast a higher vegetable content and therefore fill you up with fibre, making you feel full more quickly.

Steer clear of: Poppadoms. The world's most moreish crisps are deep fried and very porous. Try a spicy chapati instead.

CHINESE

Take the favourite: A lot of Chinese food is deep-fried in vegetable oil. The trouble begins with preparation. In a beef stir-fry for instance, the meat is half-cooked in oil before being thrown into the wok. So although the stir-fry itself boasts little oil, the meat is already saturated with it. Also, Chinese food is usually a shared experience where too many dishes are ordered and portion distortion comes into play. So start with small offerings and have a second helping only if you feel hungry. Choose bean curd, fish, shrimp, steamed ribs and chicken dishes.

Steer clear of: Batter-fried foods, sweet and sour dishes and sweet duck sauce.

PIZZA

Take the favourite: Take a thin-based pepperoni pizza and you will digest 785 calories along with 35 grams of fat. And that's before a side order of garlic bread. It's the fatty meat that does it. The secret is to go for a pizza with a lean meat topping such as ham, chicken, tuna or just tomatoes. The trend towards choosing your own topping can be a real plus point for dieters, as you can add or takeaway ingredients to suit your taste or your calorie count.

Steer clear of: Deep pans and stuffed crusts.

THAI

Take the favourite: Thailand is not an overweight nation and that's not surprising when you consider their food. It's light on fats, as most dishes are either stir fried, steamed or marinated, apart from dishes made with coconut milk (it's loaded with calories). Rice and noodles are the culinary staples to which you can add fish, chicken and vegetables.

Steer clear of: Peanut sauce and curries loaded with coconut milk.

FISH AND CHIPS

Take the favourite: The great British tradition of battered cod and chips comes in at 860 calories with 44 grams of fat. But battered cod with two thirds of the batter removed, along with a smaller portion of chips and a side serving of mushy peas, brings it down to 620 calories and 24 grams of fat and makes for an excellent supper.

Steer clear of: Battered sausages and anything frittered.

A Diner's Survival Guide

★ Be smart about picking your restaurant. Choose one that offers healthy menu options. That way you can enjoy yourself without becoming fixated about calories.

★ Be aware of pre-dinner drinks. Just one alcoholic drink can loosen your inhibitions and encourage you to order higher calorie meals later on. Arrive fashionably late so you drink at the table along with a meal instead of at the bar.

★ Don't load up on bread before the meal is served. A small roll has around 84 calories – but who sticks at one? Add butter and you're climbing to over 250 calories.

★ Don't be intimidated out of making special requests. If you want the dressing on the side, ask for it. It's one of the most diet-smart choices you can make.

★ You don't have to bypass the dessert menu altogether, just make wise choices. Go for baked apples, poached pears or sorbets.

★ Portions are normally oversized at restaurants, so share a starter or a pudding with your guest.

★ Beware of words such as 'Alfredo', 'crispy', 'crunchy', 'pan-fried', 'rich', 'sautéed', 'buttery' and 'breaded' – all suggest lots of fat. 'Steamed', 'grilled', 'poached', 'flame-seared', 'broiled', 'baked' and 'blanched' are healthier eating options.

Eat your way to endless energy

If energy could be bottled then it would be a huge seller. Being tired all the time (TATT) is a 21st-century disease. Yet for many of us the going, going, gone of our get and-up-and-go is regarded as normal.

Ask yourself when was the last time you really sprang out of bed in the morning or had a naughty twinkle in your eye? If it was too long ago to remember, then you need to seriously recharge. And you know what? Simply drinking more water or slightly making over your diet could resolve your own personal energy crisis. Here are a few suggestions for powering up.

ENERGISING FOR YOUR AGE

Just like our hair, skin and make-up, our dietary needs evolve throughout our life. This all adds up to some very specific guidelines. Reach for the star nutrients that will benefit both your health and energy levels.

Twenties

You're busy building up your career, working long hours and your social life is hot to trot. Vitamin C should be your top priority. Smoking, alcohol overload, fast-food addiction and burning the candle at both ends can all take their toll. Vitamin C is a powerful antioxidant and is involved in a large number of biological processes, which is why it's essential for health. It also helps your body to absorb iron and folic acid effectively and turn food into energy. Deficiency symptoms include bleeding gums, easy bruising and frequent colds. Fresh fruit and vegetables are good sources of vitamin C, particularly tomatoes, potatoes, oranges, cabbage and peppers. And as your bones are still growing, keep them happy and strong with a calcium fix of yoghurt, tofu, cheddar cheese and sardines.

Thirties

These are your peak childbearing years, so if you're planning a mini-you, start taking folic acid (200mcg a day). That is essential for the development of a healthy baby. The B vitamins are important too. Vitamin B1 (thiamin) is needed to convert carbohydrates into energy and keep both body and mind in shape, but like vitamin C it's water soluble, so easily lost from the body. Though it's found naturally in wholegrains and brown rice, it's also wise to take supplements as well. Vitamin B2 (Riboflavin) also helps to convert food into energy and a lack of it can stop vitamin B6 from working. It helps with women who suffer from PMS and also helps regulate sex hormones. In this case, it's best to take a vitamin B multicomplex supplement, which will cover all your needs.

Forties

Low fat and high fibre should be your aim now. You don't need as many calories as you did a decade or so ago because your metabolism decreases up to 5 per cent with each decade. Regular exercise (more of which later) and a diet rich in fresh fruit, vegetables, grains, fish and lean meats will keep you on the right track to maintain high energy levels and sidestep unwanted flab.

Fifties and Beyond

Calcium and omega-3 essential fatty acids should be on your must-eat list. Your body's calcium requirement goes up upon entering the menopause and the essential fatty acids found in oily fish keep you heart healthy and your cholesterol levels down. This is a crucial time to cut back on calories and fat for positive body benefits – limiting alcohol, caffeine and spicy foods can help with hot flushes as well as keeping energy levels at a peak in these late-afternoon years.

BEATING THE ENERGY TRAPS
Dehydration

Dehydration causes your body to lose energy by decreasing blood circulation. This deprives your muscles of oxygenated blood and causes you to become tired. Even mild dehydration can make you feel sluggish. Look out for key symptoms: constipation, dry tongue and strong-smelling urine.

Beat it: Be sure to drink enough so that your urine is

constantly pale yellow in colour, and replace lost
fluids regularly during hot weather or when working
out.

A Sweet Tooth

Sugar plays havoc with your glycaemic levels and leads
to very quick highs and then incredible blood-sugar
lows (hypoglycaemia). Simple refined sugars lurking in
fizzy drinks, chocolate and cakes may well give you a
sharp energy boost but never a lasting one. These
foods trigger a large output of insulin which lowers
blood sugar and leaves you feeling slothful. It goes
without saying that you should try and cut back on
them as much as possible. Try to be aware of hidden
sugars too. Common sugar labelling includes corn
syrup, dextrose, fructose and lactose.
Beat it: Snack regularly throughout the day on fresh
fruit and raw nuts. These will provide you with stabil-
ising nutrients.

Coffee

I've already mentioned caffeine briefly in the cravings
box, but to recap further, a study found that drinking
two to three cups of coffee daily significantly
increased stress hormone levels and blood pressure.
These effects might still be present at bedtime,
preventing you from falling peacefully into the land of
sweet dreams, and so you wake up tired and low in
energy.

Beat it: If you drink coffee, try and get your fix before noon, as it can take up to 12 hours to eliminate it from your system.

A Lack of Iron

Iron is essential for the manufacture of haemoglobin, a substance that carries oxygen around the body. A deficiency of iron can lead to anaemia. Many women can suffer from an iron deficiency without really knowing it and most are at risk because of blood loss through monthly bleeding. A government report showed that 89 per cent of women aged between 19 and 50 years were consuming less than the RDA of iron – 14mg. Tiredness and lack of energy are signs that you could need a boost of iron.

Beat it: Include more iron-rich foods in your diet, including red meat, canned tuna, sardines, oysters and dried fruit, or take iron supplements.

 TIME TO DITCH *Boiling vegetables. It can reduce the iron content by 20 per cent.*

 CHANGE IT NOW *Steam vegetables in a covered pot in as little water as possible and for the shortest time.*

Taking stock of your fridge and larder

'I'm on the seafood diet. I see food and I eat it.'
Anon

The most carefully constructed get-slim-forever-plan won't work if your kitchen is always heaving with naughty-but-nice foods that can hijack your madeover nutritional plans. The idea is to have items on hand that will allow you to rustle up tasty and healthy meals.

THE WELL-STOCKED FRIDGE MUST HAVES

★ *Avocados:* Don't worry about the high fat content, it's classed as a good fat! Avocados are great as a guacamole or added to a salad.

★ *Eggs:* Scramble, poach and boil them.

★ *Fresh ginger:* For meat, fish or vegetable dishes.

★ *Frozen peas (in the freezer):* Add to risottos, pasta sauces and vegetable curries.

★ *Lemons:* Squeeze over fish.

★ *Natural yoghurt:* Use to add depth to curries or for marinades on meat.

★ *Parmesan:* Sprinkle over a tomato-based pasta to give

instant sophistication and taste. Try it with beans on toast too.

★ *Red peppers:* Higher in beta-carotene than the other colours and great for roasting or using with dips instead of pitta bread.

★ *Smoked salmon:* Add to scrambled eggs or use in sandwiches for essential fish oils.

★ *Soups:* Ideally fresh and not tinned, they're great for a late-night supper along with some tasty bread and a small piece of cheese.

★ *Spinach (in the freezer):* Teeming with iron, this is good in curries, with eggs or as a nutritious side dish.

★ *Prepared chicken or turkey:* If you like to eat meat but want to avoid the processed stuff like cold cuts, buy it precooked and slice it into a salad or pasta dish.

★ *Tomatoes:* You can never have too many of these. Grill them or use them in salads and sandwiches or just pop them into your mouth on their own. Little cherry tomatoes make for a great TV snack.

★ *Tomato-based pasta sauces or passata:* Told you you can't get enough tomatoes! Use them in pasta or spaghetti dishes or casseroles along with fresh herbs such as basil.

Things to avoid: Pizza and garlic bread in the freezer. These make for very tempting easy meals, but they're full of saturated fat.

TIME TO DITCH *Becoming a fridge-food magnet.*

 CHANGE IT NOW *The food in your fridge is perishable. So make sure you don't find yourself eating them all just to beat the use-by date.*

THE WELL-STOCKED LARDER MUST HAVES

★ *Capers:* To add instant zing to salads, dressings, fish and meat dishes.

★ *Carrots:* Great for a healthy crunch factor when a snack attack strikes and also good for throwing into stews and soups.

★ *Dried wholemeal pasta and brown long-grain or wild rice:* Both have a good glycaemic index rating, which helps minimise swings in blood-sugar levels.

★ *Tinned pulses:* Including cannelloni, red kidney beans and butter beans. Add to salads, soups and risottos to increase the fibre content of the meal.

★ *Extra virgin olive oil:* For roasting vegetables, making salad dressing and frying onions and garlic for sauces.

★ *Jars of pesto:* It gives the necessary kick to pasta dishes.

★ *Tinned baked beans:* For a quick lunchtime filler on toast.

★ *Mustard:* Lower in fat than mayonnaise and delivers more 'guts' to sandwiches.

★ *Oats:* High in calcium and fibre. Make them into an enjoyable steaming bowl of porridge.

★ *Onions and garlic:* The staples of all kinds of sauces, soups and plenty of other dishes, these two rescue many a meal from boredom.

★ *Stock cubes:* For stock, obviously.
★ *Sweet potatoes:* The sweet orange-fleshed tatty is higher in beta-carotene than the white one and also offers vitamin C, potassium and fibre. Just make sure you eat the skin.

Things to avoid: Sugary cereals. They are often little healthier than sweets and biscuits.

ID YOUR FRIDGE (THEN MAKE IT OVER)

'Stressed spelled backwards is desserts. Coincidence? I think not.'

Unknown

The Fats Fridge

Contents: Ice cream, full-fat milk, yoghurts, beef, salad dressings, full-fat cheeses, bacon.

Nutritional makeover: Wow! This fridge is fat central. Replace the ice-cream, regular yoghurt and mayonnaise with low-fat or non-fat versions. The same goes for the milk and cheese. Edam and cottage cheese are good choices. Be aware of mayonnaise-based items like potato salad. In general, the creamier the product, the higher the fat content. Tomato-based items like salsa will be much lower in fat. White meat can be used instead of ground beef. And grill the bacon before adding it to a baguette along with lettuce and tomato (no mayo to keep the fat count down).

The Junk Food Fridge

Contents: Burgers, oven-ready chips, microwave meals, pizza, cold cuts, cheesecake.

Nutritional makeover: This fridge is loaded with high-fat, high-salt, high-sugar and zero-protein foods. It's craving for more complex carbohydrate foods like beans, fruit, vegetables and wholegrain bread. Swap chips for jacket potatoes, cheesecake for sorbets and pizza for grilled tomatoes on wholemeal bread along with olives. Microwave meals are fine when time is tight, but not as a regular substitute for home-made food. As a rough guide, look for options that contain less than 10g sugar, 20g fat and 5g saturated fat.

The Empty Fridge

Contents: A nail polish and lipstick (well, their formulas do keep better when chilled!), wine or champagne.

Nutritional makeover: This fridge says, 'I don't care about food, I just like having a good time!' Well, that's great, but when nursing a morning-after-the-night-before hangover you need good healthy basics to reach for. Frozen vegetables, bread, rice and bananas (for energy) should all be on diva standby, along with chicken and baby peeled carrots for snacks. Trade the wine and champagne in for a tomato or unsweetened fruit juices.

GET GORGEOUS: 20 INSTANT MAKEOVER NUTRITIONAL TIPS

1. Peel a banana before bed. Loaded with potassium and magnesium, this yellow wonder is high in the amino acid tryptophan, which encourages sleep.

2. Garnish with parsley. This humble herb is a natural diuretic that can help reduce that grab-the-elastic-waistband monthly bloating. The volatile oils in parsley stimulate tiny filters in your kidneys, promoting them to increase urine.

3. Get friendly with a kiwi. They contain twice the vitamin C of an orange and around four times the fibre of a stick of celery and are a good source of vitamin E and potassium.

4. Get brilliant with broccoli. Florets add the crunch in stir-fries and salads. They take just a few minutes to boil and are known to contain a special anti-cancer chemical called sulphorane.

5. Get happy with the ketchup. Lycopene is the antioxidant that gives tomatoes their bright red colour. Processed tomatoes are a better source of lycopene than raw.

6. Sex up your pizza. Next time you buy it ready-made, add an extra topping of fresh or frozen vegetables before you pop it into the oven. Sweetcorn or sliced peppers are a quick and easy way to add vitamins and fibre to your meal.

7. Trade up your bags of crisps for nuts. Unsalted nuts are a good source of protein, unsaturated fatty acids and vitamin E.

8. Let your mood be blue. For berries. Blueberries and bilberries contain anthocyanins, powerful antioxidants that are thought to boost the production of collagen to help your skin stay firm. It's also been reported that blueberries are important for improving short-term memory.

9. Live it up with live yoghurt boasting probiotics – friendly bacteria that keep your body's defences strong. Look for acidophilus and bifidis on the label to help fight against bacterial imbalance in the gut. Great for women prone to yeast infections.

10. Dunk your teabag instead of a digestive. Dipping your teabag up and down for a minute releases more of the tea's antioxidant compounds into the water.

11. Talking tea, go for green. Green tea is rich in polyphenols that fight free radicals and help prevent heart disease and cancer. It's also said to speed up your metabolic rate and therefore fight unwanted fat.

12. Think twice about eating 'slimming' foods. They're either loaded with extra sugar or simply sold in smaller portions.

13. In a hurry and need a snack? Whizz up a smoothie using a chopped banana, some fresh strawberries and a couple of tablespoons of low-fat yoghurt. Experiment with other tasty combinations.

14. Dress a bagel with raspberry jam instead of cream cheese. A published study reported that when raspberries are cooked and then preserved their antioxidant levels increase twofold.

15. Follow the good chocolate guide. White chocolate

contains more vegetable fat than cocoa, milk chocolate is slighter better for you than white and a couple of squares of dark chocolate can be more satisfying than a whole bar of the cheaper, milkier ones, due to its high percentage of cocoa solids.

16. Use peanut butter on your toast or muffin instead of butter. Peanut butter is rich in cholesterol-lowering monounsaturated fat.

17. Sweeten your tea with honey, not sugar. It's loaded with natural sugars that can boost your endurance. Why do you think bees are mad for it?

18. Don't be fooled by energy bars. Some can pack as many calories as a bar of chocolate. Look for ones that are high in fibre, low in fat and sugar, and contain ingredients such as raisins, peanuts, cereal or granola.

19. If you're a lover of creamy salad dressings, pour them onto the side of the dish and dip your fork in before stabbing your lettuce. This way you get the taste with only a fraction of the calories.

20. To lose weight, eat three apples a day. A US study found that those who munched an apple before every meal lost a stone and a half in three months. Researchers believe that this incredible weight loss is due, in part, to the fruit's skin, which contains 5g of fibre. Therefore it fills you up before your meals and helps lower cholesterol.

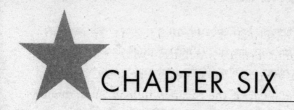

CHAPTER SIX

Your body MOT (Make Over Today)

'Physical fitness is not only one of the most important keys to a healthy body, it's the basis of dynamic and creative intellectual activity.'
John F. Kennedy

Exercise loves every body, whatever shape, size or age you are. Regular exercise promotes weight loss, increases energy and metabolism, improves strength and flexibility, decreases stress, lightens mood and helps fight disease.

You probably know a woman in your life who exercises two, three or maybe four times a week. Not only does her body look good, but she radiates inner fitness: her skin is glowing, her mood is kite-high and she's full of enthusiasm and ready to tackle anything, however busy she seems. Exercise has that effect. It's addictive. But it's not her Stairmaster or her treadmill she's hooked on, it's her chemistry. When she's exercising, her brain releases chemicals called endorphins that boost her mood and make her feel good about herself. Endorphins have a similar chemical structure to morphine and are the body's natural painkillers. They have a mild analgesic effect and they're the real reason why we should take up exercise.

But what sort of exercise? Well, just as no diet suits all, no workout fits all either. All shapes are unique, but each has the potential to be the best it can.

The key is to look at yourself, not others. Realistically assessing and accepting what you have is the way to get the most out of your fitness routine. If your physical type is naturally curvy, a lean dancer's physique will be well beyond you. Enrolling in a super-slim teacher's ballet class will not guarantee you'll emerge looking like her. And that's an important first fitness step to learn: work with your body type and not against it for your individual personal best.

This chapter isn't about out-of-this-world-workouts or how to enlist the help of a fancy trainer, it's about getting off the starting block and coming up with your own personal fitness formula.

But whatever you do, one thing's for sure: you've got to make it fun or you won't go back for seconds.

Making over your fitness attitude

So, what's stopping you from having the body you really want? Is it that you don't have time to exercise, you find it boring or you feel you can never reach your fitness ideal so don't bother even starting? Everybody faces fitness blocks – the secret is to identify them so you can break through your own personal fitness barrier.

Excuses, excuses, excuses. What's yours?

'I never have any time.'

Your get moving mindset: A little something is better than nothing at all. First off, put exercise on your weekly must-do priority list and be prepared to do exercise outside the gym. Take a pair of trainers into work and slip them on for a lunchtime power walk. Cycle into work or walk to the shops instead of driving. If you watch television, you've got time to exercise. Watch while you work out by doing some squats, crunches, tricep chair dips and bicep curls. Research shows that doing several short spurts of exercise – five, ten or fifteen minutes for a total of half an hour a day – provides as many fitness and health benefits as a single longer session.

'I can't afford a gym membership.'

Your get moving mindset: You don't even have to enter a gym to get fit. Walking or running in your nearest park is a great way to start. It's a stress-free environment and the fresh air and direct oxygen will allow you to work longer and harder. It's more strenuous than working out in a gym, so you'll burn more calories and get a better result. It's true – running on grass is 10 per cent harder than running on a treadmill.

Nothing beats jumping into your local pool for a workout either. Regular swimming is an excellent method of achieving all-round fitness as it uses all the muscle groups of the body.

As a last get-fit pay-less alternative, take inspiration from a friend of mine who bought a dog and lost pounds into the bargain with twice daily walkies!

'I'm too tired.'

Your get moving mindset: This excuse lands you in a catch 22 situation. The more sedentary you are, the more fatigued you become. And the more fatigued you are, the less exciting a workout sounds. Yet exercise makes you feel more revived than a nap and regular physical activity increases your energy. Once you get your blood flowing, a shorter workout often turns into a much longer one.

Reframe the way you think about exercise. Begin to think of it as a plus point in your life instead of another 'must', 'should' or 'ought'. And go with your moods. If you're having a low-energy day, just schedule yourself in for half an hour rather than an hour. That way you won't feel guilty if you've given up halfway through your session.

'I'm too out of shape.'

Your get moving mindset: It can be hard to don Lycra and hit the gym if you're feeling self-conscious. But gyms are full of people of all shapes and sizes and they're all there for one reason: to get fitter.

The key is to start off with baby steps, walking on the treadmill for instance. And until you gain your confidence, why not head for the gym at the times when it's not too crowded? If your day allows it, go in the afternoon, not early morning or late evening when gyms are at their busiest.

'Exercise bores me.'

Your get moving mindset: You're bored because you're stuck doing something you just don't enjoy. But exercise doesn't have to make you miserable to be worthwhile.

Figure out what's causing your boredom. Is it the place? The class you're doing? The cure may be as easy as just mixing things up a bit. If you're sitting on an indoor bike just cycling aimlessly, why not buy a mountain bike and head outside? Or take a spinning class? Involve your friends too. A Pilates class followed by a gossip in the sauna afterwards can be as much fun as having a glass of wine or two. And less calorific!

Another way to overcome boredom is to time your gym visit to coincide with your favourite TV show. It makes running on the treadmill go that much quicker.

DISCOVER YOUR WORKOUT PERSONALITY

Not getting the Goddess-like body you desire from your workout? It could be you're not tapping into your true workout personality. Get it right and you will get the most from your fitness programme. Which one are you?

Class Clubber

Extroverted, fun-loving and outgoing, you like nothing more than the buzz of the class environment to get you going and crave the company of others to stay moving. *Ways to exercise smarter:* Make working out feel like part of your social scene. Choose classes with a fast beat: salsa, step or other dance-led classes that get you fit while hooking you up with new people.

Solo and Motivated

Although you're social, when it comes to working out you prefer your own company. You're extremely self-motivated and determined to get the very best from the time you invest in the gym.
Ways to exercise smarter: Don't forget fitness should be fun. Trade some of your no-frills exercise sessions in for something exciting like a martial arts class. And keep your programme varied. Remember variety will stop your muscles from getting bored.

Social Butterfly

In the gym, just as your social life, you love flitting about, never staying on one piece of equipment for very long.

Ways to exercise smarter: Variety is great in a workout, but being too flighty with your routine will not give your body the chance to reap any benefits. Classes are the best option for you, as you have to stay the full session!

Stressed Suit

You have limited time to get fit. You have the schedule from hell and need a rapid but functional workout. *Ways to exercise smarter:* Use the 'total body' fitness equipment such as cross trainers that work both your upper and lower body at the same time. Also take up yoga or Tai Chi to help ease your stress!

Lessons from successful exercisers

'I'm in shape. Round is a shape, isn't it?'
Anon

There's no denying the rush of pure adrenaline when you first start an exercise programme. You're brimming with pumped-up enthusiasm and eager to see the transformation of flab into toned muscle. Three months down the line your enthusiasm has withered and even though you're feeling better, that fitness miracle you so eagerly anticipated hasn't quite happened. You're now in pole position to become the next exercise dropout. A conservative estimate is that at least half of exercisers drop out within the first two to three months.

Sports psychologists state that how you exercise has as much to do with your head as your body. Motivation has to be personal. It's been typically found that people driven by self-determination and personal motives are more likely to achieve success. Getting and keeping fit is a quest for personal development and empowerment, so highly successful exercisers are always pushing themselves and learning something new about their bodies – how muscles should feel and work when flexed for instance. It's how professional athletes work.

Getting into shape can be tough, but staying with your exercise regime can be even harder. So to re-energise fed-up bodies, here are the tested and sometimes surprising tactics that professionals and dedicated exercisers use. I hope they will help turn your going-nowhere routine into a programme that will not only get you moving but challenge you too.

SET GOALS

Setting goals from the outset is paramount. Ideally they should be achievable but challenging. One of the main reasons people become demotivated is because they have too high expectations of themselves. When they don't see results in a couple of weeks, they take a step back and start losing interest.

So have a purpose as your starting-point. If you're aiming to fit into a wedding dress by the summer, for example, then that's your self-confessed purpose. And if you don't have exact aspirations, put on a too tight pair of jeans, then try them on every week and be motivated by how much looser they feel.

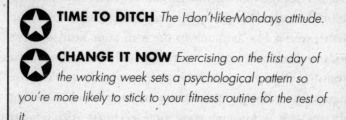

★ **TIME TO DITCH** *The I-don't-like-Mondays attitude.*

★ **CHANGE IT NOW** *Exercising on the first day of the working week sets a psychological pattern so you're more likely to stick to your fitness routine for the rest of it.*

MOVE ON FROM WEIGHT LOSS

Measuring your success by weight loss alone is not an accurate way of measuring your progress. If you are losing fat but gaining muscle, it can make it seem like you're not getting anywhere. This is why I chucked out the scales years ago.

Also, it's healthier to focus on improving your cardiovascular fitness rather than dropping the pounds. Researchers have found that having a moderate to high fitness level resulted in a 43 to 52 per cent reduced risk of death from heart disease or cancer, regardless of your body mass index. In other words, your fitness level is more important than your body fat percentage when it comes to avoiding certain health problems.

Weight loss is a welcome by-product of exercise, of course. But think of progress as maybe walking 20 minutes longer than you did five weeks ago or lifting heavier dumbbells than you did three months ago. If you keep exercising you'll be making progress even if the scales aren't reflecting it.

TALK TO YOURSELF

No, it's not the first sign of fitness madness! Motivational self-talk really does produce better performances. Sticking with exercise has as much to do with your head as your body and self-talk is a motivational tool that can be taken from the Olympic track into your own workout. Personal mantras have been proven to be a driving force. Heartening phrases such as 'Looking good' or 'I feel great – this is what I've been striving for' can be used when fatigue sets in.

INVEST IN NEW EQUIPMENT

You know the feeling when you buy a new dress and you just want to slip it on and show it off? Well, the same works for a new pair of running shoes, a new tennis racquet or workout outfit.

When was the last time you made over your gym kit? If you've had the same pair of smelly trainers for years, chuck them out and invest in a new pair. Not only will it save your style, but it will deliver more support and comfort too. Working out in a baggy old T-shirt and shapeless tracksuit bottoms doesn't give you much incentive to hit the gym either. Get your body back on track with new kit. It really does make a big difference.

GET A PERSONAL TRAINER

Thanks to lower prices and an ever-growing number of certified trainers, this service is now no longer for the elite. And there are many benefits to having a trainer. No matter what fitness level you're at now, a trainer can design a programme to push you that little bit further. They will also teach you about your muscles and emphasise the importance of warming up and stretching out – two vital steps self-exercisers usually skip to save time.

If you haven't got the budget to go one on one, you can share sessions with friends. That can keep the price per workout down to about the cost of a cinema ticket. Or you could schedule appointments less often. You don't have to work out with a trainer once a week to see results – take their knowledge and check in once a month with them. Or, if you're really dedicated, you could book block trainer sessions. That way you would usually get a discount.

BANISH ROUTINE

OK, I know I have used the word 'routine' here, but for constant stimulation your workout routine should be anything but. Doing the same thing over and over again until your body feels as though it's on a hamster wheel is not a good thing. People who've been successful at losing weight or changing their body composition never stick with the same workout for long, they're constantly re-evaluating it. It can be little things such as running at a faster speed or putting the treadmill on an incline, but the idea is to mix up your workout and cross-train as much as possible. Surprise your body every time you take it out to be exercised.

Exercises That Deliver the Fastest Results

★ **Interval training.** In simple terms that's taking it fast and then taking it slow. It fights off boredom and efficiently combines aerobics with conditioning, giving the body the best of both worlds in the shortest possible time. For example in half an hour you could include 10 minutes on the bike, 10 lunges, 10 half press-ups, 10 minutes running on the treadmill, 10 squats and 10 tricep dips, then round it off with abdominal exercises.

★ **Walking at a constant brisk pace.** This adds up to an aerobically challenged workout which tones and strengthens the whole body, especially the legs and bottom, without adding bulk. Stride out for at least 20 minutes three to five times a day – if pushed for time, aim for 10 minutes in the morning and 10 minutes in the evening walking at 3 mph. As a rough guideline that's enough to make you breathe more heavily but still be able to carry on a conversation.

Fitness by numbers

Scientists are finding that the body ages faster if you don't exercise. Studies show that conditions we attribute to ageing, such as weight gain, weakness, stiffness and bone loss, can be slowed or even reversed with resistance training. It's no exaggeration to say that a 40-year-old who exercises frequently can have the body age of a 30-something.

The key to biological clock-stopping is to let exercise evolve over the decades. It's not so much what you do, it's the mix of activities over time that is important, together with the constant maintenance of fitness levels.

If you've been neglecting your body, take heart, it's never too late to start being physically active (after a consultation with your GP), but you must stick with it. Here is a simple exercise programme for each decade.

TWENTIES

If you're exercising now you are helping to increase your longevity and decreasing your risk of disease. Not that you're worried about this now, your top priority is looking good! But if you achieve optimum fitness now you can coast off that hard work well into your thirties.

Your weekly workout guide: Your heart and lung capacity

allows you to exercise aerobically for longer now, so make the most of sports games along with friends, slotting in at least 20–30 minutes of cardio activity three times a week.

These are also the years for peak bone mass, so step up on resistance training with dumbbells to work the upper body and swimming to help with the lower body.

Try and maintain a healthy weight – if you need to lose it, do it, as it will be easier now than ever. Research shows that after the age of 30 lean body mass and metabolic rate decline.

But although you may be raring to go, be careful not to burn out. Take days off in between workouts for the body to rest and build muscle. And be realistic about your goals: aiming for a weight that's too low can be hazardous to your health.

THIRTIES

You're probably working harder and longer than ever before and may have the added responsibility of a family. But if you're ever going to train hard, now is the time to do it. These are the years when you'll really be able to maximise your intensity and endurance abilities. And the harder you train, the more easily you'll be able to prevent the natural fat gain and muscle loss that will happen unless you do something about it.

Your weekly workout guide: Increase your cardiovascular output. Start with three 20-minute sessions a week. That sounds a lot but it can be incidental exercise – that's unplanned, gym-free activity such as climbing the stairs, walking and vigorous housework. It's all exercise, whether it's working out in the gym or washing the car. You may also want to strength train your weak spots such as the abdominals, chest and lower and upper back.

Make your weekends count too: if you've got the time, slot in some press-ups, lunges and sit-ups or take a cycle ride with the kids. And try and see exercise as a treat rather than a hardship. It will do wonders for your motivation.

FORTIES

Although it's said that socially the forties are the new thirties, realistically you're a mid-lifer with a potential body crisis. As weight settles on around the hips, stomach and upper arms, your natural reaction is to panic diet. Initially, after promising results, a self-defeating cycle of yo-yo dieting can kick in and before you know it you're depleting your body of lean muscle mass.

Your weekly workout guide: Strength is crucial to help replace lost muscle, get the body's metabolism back up and keep weight off permanently. Aim to do five training sessions within a two-week period, with one or two days off in between sessions. Add a good dose of cardio too. Choose an activity that's not too joint-jarring and that you enjoy doing.

Time and money are usually a little generous during this decade, so why not enlist the help of a personal trainer to kickstart a stale routine?

FIFTIES AND BEYOND

This is the time you've got to exercise for your health without overdoing it. Many people get to this age and become extremely unfit and very weak because of lack of movement and age-related muscle loss. If you're just picking up exercise after a very long sabbatical, don't start acting like a 20-something just because you feel energised. Take it slowly. A complete physical might even be necessary. *Your weekly workout guide:* Start with half an hour twice a week, whether it's walking, a beginner's aerobics class or swimming, which is especially good as it places less stress on the skeletal system, as weight is supported by the water. All these forms of exercise will raise the heart rate and help to reduce hardening of the arteries. Working with light weights is good, as older muscle responds to training by getting stronger and leaner. To enhance flexibility, do some stretching exercises daily. Keep abreast of new trends – classes aren't just for the young and Pilates and Tai Chi are both recommended for those in these decades, so check out your local leisure centre.

★ **TIME TO DITCH** *Doing the easy stuff first.*

★ **CHANGE IT NOW** *Reverse your cardio workout. Do the sweaty stuff first then ease into the moderate exercise. This can burn as much as 3 per cent more fat yet makes your exercise session feel less like an endurance test.*

Steps to a faster metabolism

Metabolism: it's the chemical process by which our body breaks down food to produce energy and it has a direct bearing on how much we can eat without gaining weight.

Let's face it, some people are just born lucky and blessed with a fast metabolism which allows them to burn calories faster and eat more than their fair share of chocolate cake. Don't you just hate them?

But rather than cursing your slow metabolic rate, you would do better to admire the efficiency with which the body manages the ups and downs of its energy needs and learn how to work with it rather than against it.

 TIME TO DITCH *Bland food.*

 CHANGE IT NOW *Livening up your food with spices such as cayenne pepper, ginger root and chilli peppers can give your metabolism a boost.*

A woman's metabolism, like everything in life, changes with age, with most of us experiencing a 5 to 10 per cent drop in our metabolic rate every decade. This can result in an average gain of five pounds every ten years. In your happy I-can-eat-all-I-want twenties, your metabolism is at its peak, largely because the two key factors that determine it – muscle mass and hormone levels – are also at their highest and most efficient. Hit your thirties and your metabolism rate is telling a different story. The numbers are creeping up on the scale as metabolism naturally declines and weight-bearing exercise takes a back seat.

Now what's going on in your forties? This is when muscle loss really starts to kick in. Beginning with this decade, most women lose about one third of a pound of muscle a year and as you enter the peri-menopausal stage (roughly the 15 years leading up to the menopause), changes in hormones shift fat storage and you begin to experience what is called middle age spread around the stomach.

So, the question you're begging to ask is what can you do to speed your metabolism up? Well, quite a lot actually. The good news is that the factors that affect this biochemical process are not beyond your control and now you've (hopefully) mapped out your fitness plan, you can set to work on putting those suggestions in action, along with a few others, to become an efficiently fuelled fat-burning machine.

Rather than list a rigid set of rules to improve your metabolism, I decided a more friendly way would be to map out a way you can start making over your metabolism in a day. Here it is:

Your Daily Metabolism Makeover

7 a.m. Rise and shine. Getting up an hour earlier than usual every day can burn off extra calories. Carrying out light household chores can use up 2.2 times your basal metabolic rate (BMR) – that's an extra 75 calories burned on top of your BMR per hour. Take note: your BMR is the lowest number of calories you need daily for your body to carry out basic automatic functions.

8 a.m. Breakfast like a king. A light meal including some protein, carbohydrate and fat (poached eggs on toast with a sprinkling of nuts for example) is the ideal combination to avoid hunger pangs later in the morning. A cup of coffee with your breakfast will increase alertness and boost metabolism.

9 a.m. Hot foot it to work. Swap your train commute for a walk to work – even if it's just part of the way. This will help convert the carbohydrate in your breakfast to glycogen (starch) for your muscle stores and will give your metabolic rate a boost as well as eating up about 3.5 times the calories of your normal BMR.

10 a.m. Drink water. When the body is parched it often transmits hunger signals and dehydration can also lead to a sluggish metabolism. Also, if you're deskbound, start fidgeting. For every hour of moving around you can use up an extra 50 calories or more, depending on your BMR.

11 a.m. Eat a small snack. Eating frequent, small

and nutritious snacks four to six times a day keeps
your metabolism rate 'revved' up all day long.

12 a.m. Chill a little. And prepare your digestive
system for lunch. It will absorb food better if you are
not tense.

1–2 p.m. Get adequate protein from your lunch.
Your body uses about 20 to 30 per cent more energy to
digest protein than to digest carbs or fat. A protein-led
salad of chicken with a little brown rice for instance will
also help combat a post-lunch slump in energy.

3–4 p.m. Shave your sugar intake. This is the
most common time to be reaching for an energy
booster in the form of sugary snacks. But too much
sugar causes your insulin levels to soar, which tells
your body to stop metabolising and start storing fat.
Have healthy snacks instead.

5–6 p.m. Hit the gym. The American Council on
Exercise reveals that studies have consistently shown
that exercising during these hours produces better
performance and more power. Muscles are warm and
more flexible, strength is at its peak and resting heart
rate and blood pressure are low.

7–8 p.m. Modify happy hour. Those who combine
alcohol and high-fat foods burn fewer calories and
store more fat. Instead, head home and prepare a
nutritious meal – but don't skimp on calories.
Radically reducing caloric intake causes the body to
hold onto stored calories and that can slow metabolism by as much as 30 per cent.

9 p.m. Calm down. According to Dr Pamela Peeke, author of *Fight Fat after Forty* (Piatkus Books), stress causes an increase in the hormone cortisol, which in turn boosts cravings for carbs and fats. Deep breathing exercises will help the body relax.

10–11 p.m. Check in for sleep. A study from the University of Chicago found that just one week of sleep deprivation encourages the body to overproduce insulin, which increases the tendency to store fat. Also, when you're tired you have less energy for extra calorie-burning activities the next day. Try and get at least seven hours of sleep every night.

Get on a higher plane and makeover your mind

'Tension is who you think you should be. Relaxation is who you are.'
Dorothy Parker

Higher, higher, higher ... if that's the way your stress levels are going, you're more than likely to eat more, exercise less and feel downright moody.

Stress has been billed as the epidemic of the 21st century. And in a way it is. Fifty years ago only bridges were stressed – humans were nervous, anxious or worried! But today stress is seemingly linked with virtually every human misery.

 TIME TO DITCH *Thinking 'What went wrong today?'*

 CHANGE IT NOW *Think: 'What went right today?'*

But before I go on about coping with it, let's hear some

good news about being stressed. Yes, there is some! We all need a certain amount of hassles a day to keep us ticking over. It would hardly be worth getting out of bed if we didn't have some pressures to motivate us. It is a fact that increased stress results in increased productivity – up to a point. However, this level differs for each of us. It's very much like a stress on a guitar string – not enough produces a dull, raspy sound, too much makes a shrill, annoying noise, but just the right amount can create high-performing tones. Similarly, we all need to find a healthy stress level.

Are You Addicted to Stress?

We have become a generation of compulsive busy-bodies and to say you aren't stressed is almost to admit you're a failure. Why? Because your life isn't busy enough! Crazy, eh? Competitive stress syndrome is on the rise, so be honest and ask yourself why you like to be seen as addicted to drama. Could it be that:

★ It helps you seem important and indispensable.
★ It helps you avoid responsibility. Obviously you're too stressed to be given more work or chores!
★ It helps you maintain a distance. Anyone as important as you can't be expected to indulge in idle chit-chat!
★ It gives you a chemical high. You've become addicted to your own adrenaline.
★ It helps you avoid success. Why risk rising up the

> ladder when by simply saying you're stressed you
> can avoid it all?
> ★ You don't have to seen as having a sense of
> humour. Stress is no laughing matter and it gets
> you off the hook of having to make it one.

THE CHILL OUT PLAN WITH MINUTES TO SPARE

One of the annoying things about reading pieces on how to destress is the suggestion of taking yourself off to some swanky health spa for a week. For starters, who can afford it on a regular basis? And secondly, when do we ever get the time? Unless you're a cash-rich woman with no responsibilities, this suggestion is really just a dream.

Women today are right up against a host of new pressures that leave them feeling that they're juggling a dozen balls up in the air. If, say, a button has fallen off your jacket just in time for an important meeting and your two-year-old is throwing a tantrum as you're leaving the house, you're more than likely to be suffering from lifestyle stress. Although it's not the 'big stuff', all this 'small stuff' shouldn't be underestimated. Smaller things can build up, creating layer upon layer of strain. You may not even realise it's happening until something occurs that really makes you want to explode.

And the silly thing is, more often than not we stress ourselves out by trying to be perfect. Are you guilty of slaving away making home-made food every day instead of cheating now and again and plumping for a takeaway? Or laboriously ironing the bedsheets just because your mother did? Get a life, woman! Our downfall is that genetically we are programmed to nurture everyone else first and ourselves last. But ultimately we have to challenge where our beliefs come from and ask ourselves: 'Does this belief make life better?' If it doesn't, get rid of it.

To ease yourself calmly into your day or out of it, the secret is to arm yourself with a handful of quick rechargers that will help you to feel on top of things at any time.

If You Have 5 Minutes ... Stretch Out

Stretching can be just the tonic you need to recharge your batteries and ease down those high and tight shoulders.

To start, sit on the floor with your legs crossed comfortably in front of you and hands on your knees or in your lap. Then take a slow deep breath. Gently curve your spine and neck forward so that your spine forms a C shape as you exhale. Breathe in as you resume your starting position. Repeat this move up to 20 times. The more slowly you take it, the more it will warm up those clenched muscles in your neck and back.

If You Have 10 Minutes ... Breathe Easy

Breathing may sound easy – it's hardly an Olympic sport – but few of us actually do it properly and stress can't be managed efficiently unless you do. If you watch a baby who hasn't yet developed lazy breathing habits you will notice that their breathing is deep and their stomach visibly moves slowly up and down. This is diaphragmatic breathing – the natural way to do it.

For the ultimate calming breath try this approach: lie

down and place a large book on your stomach. On inhalation, the book should rise and on exhalation it should fall. Take ten minutes to do this and during this time take your mind off somewhere relaxing.

If You Have 15 Minutes ... Rub Tensions Away

It's no secret that one of the best weapons against stress is a massage session. When essential oils are worked into the skin something wonderful happens: they trigger responses in the brain through receptors in the nose and pores and the brain then signals various organs to produce chemicals that work on the body in specific ways.

The shoulders and feet are two areas that you can massage yourself and can be covered in just 15 minutes. Rub a couple of drops of lavender oil into a carrier oil such as almond and begin by using soothing strokes around your shoulder blades, picking up and squeezing the top of the shoulder muscles from the shoulder edge along to the neck. As for feet, don't get scientific about it, just do whatever feels good.

If You Have 30 Minutes ... Soak Away the Blues

Making over your mind can start with the smaller things in life such as sinking into a warm tub full of bubbles or mineral salts. Steal half an hour away from your normal routine and give yourself time to 'steep' yourself properly and gather your thoughts. Make it a luxury too: as well as filling up the bath with deliciously scented bubbles or lacing the water with aromatherapy oils, light scented candles and even sip a glass of wine to really wind you right down.

GET GORGEOUS: 20 INSTANT BETTER BODY TRICKS

1. Wear a sports bra. There's no point having a great body with breasts heading southwards through lack of support!

2. Insure yourself against MTV injury. At the gym, position yourself right in front of the TV screen when on your piece of equipment. This way you won't end up with your neck strained.

3. Get desk fit. To tighten your bottom while sitting at a desk, sit up straight with your feet flat on the floor and concentrate on clenching those buttocks. Hold for a few seconds, relax and repeat 20 times.

4. Literally shake off tension. When you feel your shoulders rising, shake your arms and legs loosely for a few minutes. The physical movement of getting jiggy releases stress.

5. Hate the gym? Then take up dance. Salsa, Lindy Hop, jazz and even belly dancing are structured with exact steps but are all fun forms of exercise.

6. A surefire slouch buster is to stick a pillow behind your lower back when sitting for an extended time. It helps maintain the lumbar curve (the lower part of your spine) and keeps your shoulders up.

7. Although it's not advisable to wear heels all the time, walking in them trains your legs to produce muscle, especially in the calves and thighs. When you're wearing heels, it amounts to a full day's worth of calf raises.

8. Adopt TV fitness. Move away from the sofa and sit on

a stability or Swiss ball when watching television. This way all your core muscles (the ones that give the body a corset effect) are constantly engaged, as you have to keep rebalancing yourself to stay on the ball.

9. Clip on a pedometer and aim for 10,000 steps a day to really shape up.

10. Pelvic floor exercises aren't just for post-natal women Let me be frank: doing these will not only stop you involuntary wetting yourself when laughing or coughing, but they will also work your deep abdominal muscles to great effect. Contract the muscles that you use to stop the flow of urine and hold for four to five seconds. Repeat as many times as you can throughout the day.

11. Choose fitness to suit your mood. If you feel angry, hook up with a kick-boxing class; if stressed, try yoga; if indecisive, try power walking to clear your head.

12. When gym shopping, look round for one with a pool and a sauna so you can reward yourself after working out.

13. After a satisfying workout, jot down how good you feel. Use it as a reference the next time you don't want to go.

14. Power up your stair climb. Forget looking ladylike – take your stairs two at a time and you'll target your glutes even more.

15. Get into kids' play. When hanging out at the park with friends or kids, don't just sit on the sidelines lost in thought, play Frisbee – it eats up to 350 calories an hour. Delight kids by spinning the roundabout really

hard to work chest muscles and give your toddler hard and constant pushes on the swing to firm your arms.

16. Fall into relationship fitness. Instead of sitting in a restaurant or the cinema, plan a fitness date with your guy. It's even said that those who work out together stay together!

17. Change your workout at least every 10 sessions so your body doesn't get too well-rehearsed and reach a plateau. Even just changing the order of the exercises and throwing in a couple of new ones can make a big difference.

18. While you brush your teeth, limber up by doing pliés by the sink.

19. Have a baby and no time for planned exercise? No problem. Take up buggy fitness. Stoll out with your stroller three or four times a week. Start with 20-minute walks and work up to 45-minute sessions.

20. Put a mini trampoline on your shopping list. Not only are they great fun, but 10 minutes of bouncing can benefit the body as much as 30 minutes of jogging, so they are a great investment for anyone pushed for time.

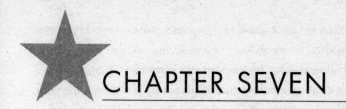

CHAPTER SEVEN

Making over your style

'Fashion is architecture. It's a matter of proportions.'
Coco Chanel

Are you a fearless follower of fashion? A fashion trooper? Or just plain unfashionable? If thinking what to wear every morning has become a trial and the last thing on your mind is retail therapy, then this chapter is just for you.

Perhaps the word 'fashion' actually scares you a little? You don't want to be a fashion victim. Perhaps the word 'style' sounds, well, more stylish, do-able and wearable?

However you prefer to describe it, I think life is too short not to dress well and there's simply no excuse for it. Slobbing about the house in old baggy T-shirts will do nothing for your get-up-and-go.

Whether you've got a high-flying job, work from home or run a household, I feel that tasks are approached with a more positive attitude if you're dressed for them. As a freelance writer I know if I get up and slip on a pair of tracksuit bottoms (that should never have come out of my gym bag) I am likely to just sink into the sofa, drink tea and munch on biscuits for most of the day. Now if I get up and dress like I mean business – and that doesn't mean an eighties-style padded shoulder suit but a great pair of jeans worn with a plain but sexily cut shirt – it instantly makes me feel on top of things and in control.

Every woman owes herself the right of dressing with style and giving yourself over to frumpiness shouldn't be an option.

The secret to pulling off desirable style is simple knowing what suits you and what most definitely doesn't. Women who have great wardrobes aren't born into them (unless they're a relative of Stella McCartney), they just know what they want and where to get it. And it's nothing to do with a generous bank balance – even the thrifty can look stylish – just about shopping super-smart.

And with great style comes great confidence. If you feel good in what you're wearing, you'll instantly shine when you enter a room. With a new pair of shoes and a great outfit, you'll feel you can go anywhere, say anything and do anything!

Are you stuck in a style rut?

So where are you now? Do you look into a wardrobe that's heaving with garments and declare you have nothing to wear? Then you're probably stuck in your very own style rut.

Being stuck in a fashion rut is rather like being stuck in a make-up rut. You always feel one giant step behind everybody else. Fashion can be challenging, so what woman hasn't wished at some point for some kind of fairy-style mother to fly in, fling open their closet and identify the strengths and weaknesses of their wardrobe?

But becoming your own closet consultant isn't such a big deal. It's not about slavishly following trends, wearing designer clothes or shopping until you drop, it's about asking yourself certain questions whenever you shop, being aware of what's happening on the catwalk, dressing for your shape, size and age (more of which later) and ultimately building up a wardrobe that passes the style test every time.

I know that not everyone likes shopping for clothes, but who doesn't like to look glamorous and get noticed? Well, your clothes can do that for you.

Apart from all this, a closet update can put a fresh spin on your attitude. I know two women who swapped their wardrobes for a week for a magazine article. The divorced mother of one who had forgotten her feminine side and ran around in jeans and flat shoes all day declared her days of being a 'boring mum' were well and truly over once she experienced the school run in heels. 'My walk took on a slight wiggle,' she said. 'The funny thing is, fashion is infectious. Several mums followed suit and started dressing up instead of down too.' Then there was the advertising executive who was always trussed up in suits and smart dresses and thought she would look too 'sloppy' in loose-cut trousers and unstructured jackets but was surprised that she could still look smart. The biggest surprise of all was that men approached her more often! 'Perhaps they were previously put off because I looked too brisk and ladylike,' she commented. Whatever, both women discovered a style side they hadn't tapped into before and now effortlessly mix their two styles.

So, let's cut to the chase and put your wardrobe on trial.

Clues Your Wardrobe is in Crisis

★ You wear the same 'best' trousers and top whether you have an important meeting at work or an evening do.

★ There are clothes in your wardrobe that you've never worn or, worse, don't remember buying.

★ The only dress-me-down clothes you own are jeans and T-shirts.

★ You only buy grey, black and white, as they're classic shades.

★ Several (okay, all) of your items bring back memories: the outfit you wore for your best friend's wedding (eight years ago), your first job interview after baby number two (10 years ago) and the outfit you met your husband in (15 years ago).

★ You frequently pass over garments because they're missing buttons, the hem is falling down, there's a stain or they need pressing.

★ You cannot pull a fabulous outfit together double quick when pressed for time.

★ You always turn down last-minute dinner-party invitations, as you have no special outfits.

★ You have yet to discover the nip-and-tuck of tailoring. Many of your clothes are shapeless to hide a multitude of sins.

★ Your wardrobe is full of make-do pieces rather than must-have pieces

If most of this is you, then you need to do more than make over your wardrobe, you need to give it a facelift! It's time to wave farewell to those 'classic' sweaters that you bought with your first pay cheque – unless, of course, they're Dior or Chanel, classed as vintage and double up as your pension.

Start treating your wardrobe as an investment, not a visual photograph to indulge your memories. Now I'm not saying you shouldn't hang onto your wedding dress or something that's truly sentimental, but if you're not wearing it, bag it up and store it rather than letting it take up valuable hanging space. Which leads me very nicely into my next section.

TIME TO DITCH *Being hung up about your size.*

CHANGE IT NOW *Cut the size labels out of your clothes so you don't have to be reminded if you don't want to. It's the cut of the clothes that matters, not the size.*

Give your wardrobe a workout

'I don't keep clothes. Goodbye. Moving on. I have a closet full of clothes. But it's just one closet. Otherwise, how do you select? You can't see.'
Diane Keaton

It's said that clutter stresses us out by creating visual noise. The same can be said for an overstuffed wardrobe. What you need here is an act of get-rid-of-it-all madness: a day where you dedicate yourself to dejunking your wardrobe and tackling all those sales mistakes and items you've been waiting to fit into for five years (and never will).

First up: chuck out your cowboy jacket. Remember, there's vintage and then there's fancy dress. Be firm, be ruthless and be unsentimental when it comes to garments that add decades onto your look and keep you truly buried in a style rut.

The best way to go about a serious dejunk is to strip down to your undies and try on every single garment. Yes, every single one! Look at yourself in a full-length mirror, do a couple of twirls and ask yourself: 'Does this make me look good? Does it show off my figure to its best advantage? Do I feel comfortable in it as well stylish?' If it doesn't do all three, then throw it out.

Have boxes and bags ready so that you don't end up with a heap of clothes piled up in the corner. Sort them into items for:

★ **Selling.** Although a dress may have been a one-hit wonder for you, it could be a treasured piece for someone else. There are now many dress agencies springing up, so gather together a bag of well-maintained clothes with sellability, drop it off at the shop and make some money off your old cast-offs to put towards a new-look you.

★ **Giving away.** These are the things that you bought on a fashion whim and will never wear again. Or that you bought when you were in between sizes and now don't fit.

★ **Storing.** It's not in fashion right now, but it could be in five years' time. If your gut feeling tells you not to throw it, then box it and store it.

★ **Throwing.** You've worn it to death and now it should be left to RIP. Clues that an item has reached this stage include worn fabric, small tears and bobbles (on knitwear).

If you've been dejunking properly, by the end of day you will have thrown out the shabby, the dated, the stretched and the unflattering colours. And if your once full wardrobe is now a sad collection of a dress, a coat and a couple of pairs of trousers, console yourself – the best is yet to happen. An excuse to shop will keep your image looking fresh. In my experience it's better to be without then cling onto something you know is wrong and won't suit you in a million years. Anything that makes you look frumpy, dumpy and lumpy does nothing for your sense of self and shouldn't be hanging in your wardrobe.

The Rut Factor Waits in ...
★ Baggy jumpers
★ Post-pregnancy clothes
★ Elasticated waistbands
★ Skirt hems that land right on the middle of the knee
★ Box-cut jackets
★ Jackets or dresses with any type of fringing
★ Any type of garment that shows the shape of your bottom or knees when you're not wearing it

---

BECOME YOUR OWN STYLE EDITOR

Making everyday dressing easy peasy is no picnic when you've got an unedited wardrobe, but now you've been ruthless and doubled, even trebled your wardrobe space, what should you be left with? Essentially it should be classics that you can build a new wardrobe around.

The Wardrobe Staples

★ A well-cut coat that pulls any outfit together
★ A great pair of black wide-legged trousers you can dress down with a T-shirt or dress up with a shirt

★ A single-breasted jacket nipped in at the waist that looks great either worn with jeans or trousers

★ Crew-neck sweater(s) in plain hues

★ Basic V-necked T-shirts. Cut is important. Do not keep them if they have square short sleeves (urgh!) or are square cut in the body.

★ Dark denim jeans. Jeans are an absolute basic. They can now be passed off as evening wear if teamed with a stunning sequinned top.

★ A crisp white shirt. Cut again is important, so choose a style that flatters.

★ A wrap dress. Indispensable. It looks smart and sexy in seconds.

★ A little black dress

★ A well-cut cardigan you can throw over trousers and dresses

★ A skirt that suits your shape

★ A denim jacket. Just keep your eye on the cut.

Now, generally these are the backbone of your wardrobe, but be aware of the dowdy factor. You may have a white shirt, but the style of collars changes and cuts are updated. There's no point hanging onto it because it's a shirt and it's white! Use your style antennae.

And don't fool yourself that 'timeless' means 'forever more'. It's just one of those fashion sayings that catch you out! Colours, textures and fabrics all evolve over time. When replenishing your wardrobe, keep a keen eye on magazines for ideas. You don't have to become a fashion aficionado, just gain enough knowledge to know what's in and what's out.

TIME TO DITCH *Ill-fitting clothes. There's no worse look.*

CHANGE IT NOW *Invest in the skills of a good local tailor who can lengthen, shorten, dart and cinch for a bespoke look. Sometimes it's a case of just shortening a hem an inch to turn something from drab to fab.*

ORGANISING YOUR WARDROBE

You've decluttered and restocked and you're well on your way to making over your style, now what you don't want is all that hard work going to waste in the shape of a muddled and shambolic wardrobe strategy. If you open your wardrobe doors and you can't see what you've got in an instant, then you won't end up wearing it. Here are a few guidelines:

★ Use wooden hangers (never wire, as they will ruin the shape of your clothes).

★ Hang clothes up either according to type (trousers, skirts or dresses) or by colour, so you can find something quickly.

★ Fold jumpers *à la* Benetton style in several shallow piles. Pile them too high and they will only end up tipping over.

★ Shoes are often just chucked into the bottom of the wardrobe. Either store them in their boxes in neat pairs or buy one of those calico shelf devices which has shoe compartments and hangs in your wardrobe. I always like to stuff the toes with tissue paper to keep their shape.

★ Hang belts on hooks either from the rail or from the doors.

★ Make sure your wardrobe smells nice by hanging up scented muslin bags or spritz a scarf with your favourite fragrance and tie it up.

★ If wardrobe space is tight, free it up by packing away either summer or winter clothes depending on the season. Use a suitcase or airtight storage boxes.

Getting it right

STEPS TO STRESS-FREE SHOPPING

I personally love shopping – it's in my DNA – but I have certain rules I abide by to ensure my precious shopping time is successful. I'm not saying I've never had fashion disasters, but I've learned from them – namely that if you have too many it ends up costing a small fortune. So here are a few tips I've picked up along the way.

First off, if you're looking to restock your wardrobe, the worse thing you can do is have a passive attitude to shopping. That's aimlessly wandering around department stores just buying bits and pieces that don't match up with anything else left in your wardrobe. The smartest move you can make is planning ahead. This way you don't lose control and you can head off style disasters.

1. Figure Yourself Out

> 'Say what you like about long dresses, but they cover a multitude of shin.'
>
> **Mae West**

Work out why the clothes left hanging in your wardrobe

suit you. When you wear them, what do people normally compliment you on? Is it your good legs? If it is, buy more skirts that show them off. Is it your toned and shapely arms? If so, short sleeves or close-fitting long-sleeved tops will go down well. Is it your great cleavage? Accentuate a generous bosom with flattering tops.

Consider your shape too. Pear shapes should never wear a drop waist and petite figures should wear clothing blessed with a little structure so they don't end up looking swamped. The secret is understanding your proportions – your weight versus your height or your shoulders versus your bosom. A full-length mirror is an absolute must to develop an eye for portion control.

2. Don't Shop on 'Fat' Days

You know the ones I mean – you're feeling pre-menstrual and your stomach is bloated. This is not a good time to shop, as you're not only feeling at your grumpiest – never a good omen for shopping –but some women can put on as much as 5lb when pre-menstrual. You're also in the danger zone of a PMS purchase. I don't know what happens during this time, but you can gravitate towards the most unsuitable garments thinking they look fab and a week down the line you can't understand what came over you.

3. Never Shop on a Saturday

If your soul mission is to replenish a depleted wardrobe you want to feel unhurried and relaxed. Saturday is not the day for this. The changing rooms are busy and you feel pressurised into giving up your cubicle more quickly than you would normally. Also, staff are rushed. So if your size isn't hanging up they're less likely to go into the stockroom to look for it. If you can book a day off in the week (Mondays are very quiet), then do; if not, head out early on Saturday morning and aim to finish shopping by midday, before crowds are at their largest.

4. Dress to Undress

There's nothing that puts you off trying on clothes faster than having to undo seemingly millions of buttons, wriggle out of too tight jeans and zip up boots. So if you're aiming to do a shop crawl of changing rooms, dress in clothes you can easily get on and off (including shoes). Wear plain seam-free underwear too, so that clothes are not distorted by lumps and bumps, put some make-up on and do your hair. It will help you visualise how great you can look in the clothes.

5. Ask Yourself: 'Will It Work with the Rest of my Wardrobe?'

If it goes with at least three items in your existing wardrobe, it will be a great buy. Otherwise, unless it's an amazing stand-alone piece you will wear again and again, think twice before buying it.

6. Ask Yourself: 'Can I Afford It?'

I'm not talking a £15 shirt that would be worth the price if only worn five times, I'm talking a costly item such as a coat, suit, dress or pair of trousers. The cost per wear is the deciding factor. Credit card debt is not smart, so decide whether or not an item is an investment buy. If, for instance, you buy a great trouser suit you could wear it as a suit or split it up separately and wear twice a week for the next nine months. If it's a classic style, you will probably still be wearing it two years later. Then it's a great buy and passes the reality test as well as the style test.

 TIME TO DITCH *Unplanned sales buying. Many a bargain has turned into an unworn bargain.*

CHANGE IT NOW *Cheap prices are tempting, but the question you need to ask is: 'Would I still buy it if it were full price?' If not, then pass it over.*

DRESSING FOR YOUR AGE
Twenties
This is the decade you can get away with wearing eye-popping bright and bold prints and patterns. If your legs are up for it, show them off with short skirts and long boots. Revel in the fact that this is the anything-that-goes decade – it's all about expressing yourself with fashion.

Thirties
This can be one of the sexiest decades, plus by now you're more clued up about what works best for you and have the confidence not to be dictated to by fashion. So pick what you like and leave what you don't. It can be as simple as that! Your budget is probably now healthier too, so aim for

quality and punch up the colour factor by teaming neutral colours with shoes or bags in bold hues.

Forties

By now you know who you are and clothes worn with confidence can empower your look. You can still follow trends, just don't make the mistake of dressing too young. Lamb and mutton do not want to belong in the same sentence when someone is discussing your look. Inject a little colour into your clothing – pink for instance reflects wonderfully back into the face, whereas top-to-toe black looks far too draining. Try new shapes, but be aware of anything too buttoned. Relax your style, otherwise you can wind up looking very uptight.

Fifties and Beyond

This can so easily be the chicest of decades. You can revel in a little glamour with distinguished little jackets and luxurious-looking buys such as a fabulous scarf. Keep your dressing fuss-free – bows, bustles and frills have long had their day – but go for distinguished and elegant colours.

HOW TO LOOK MODERN FOR WORK

With power dressing a thing of the past and the modern look for the office being a relaxed style, what are the new dress-for-success rules?

First, don't be fooled into thinking that your dress code doesn't matter. While work wear has never been so dress-down-Friday, it still has to cut a dash, if not exactly to crash through the glass ceiling then at least to make the right impression. Remember, clothes can mean business. Want to hear the evidence? Studies reveal that women who take care over their work appearance are perceived as being more competent than women who don't, are more likely to be promoted than women who don't and typically earn 20 per cent more than women who don't.

So, since image still plays such a vital role in today's work environment, it makes sense to polish up your appearance.

Dressing for the Part

Now we have concluded that nothing looks more tragically dated that a power suit, even if you are a CEO, but is wearing a print dress with sling-backs or a pair of jeans with trainers wrong as well? It depends where you work. If you're working in advertising or publishing, then dressing down wouldn't be frowned upon, especially when teamed with some great accessories like a scene-stealing bag or a pair of shoes, whereas a merchant banker or a doctor would need to dress more formally to convey confidence and gain respect. It always pays to fit in with the company dress code. At the end of the day it's how you perform in your job that counts, but if you're dressed well and you make a mistake you don't look half as bad!

Your Working Wardrobe

★ Relaxed separates have replaced formal suits. Wearing a jacket over a T-shirt is now seen as smart, stylish and acceptable. Tailored trousers with a polo or crew neck are just as suitable.

★ A well-cut cardigan, whether short or long and belted or not, can easily be passed off as the new jacket.

★ Dress every day as if you have a meeting (even if you haven't).

★ Dressing sexily for the office isn't a great career move.

★ Don't show any piercings (apart from your ears) at work!

★ Trade the briefcase in for a large leather tote bag. It looks far less official.

★ Add a stylish spark to your outfit with a great pair of boots or shoes. Not only will your feet look great but you'll also walk as if you mean business.

★ If you work in a young office and you're not so young yourself, don't be tempted to compete. Dress your age – but with oodles of style.

★ Learn to ad(dress) the balance. Dress more smartly than your boss and she will wonder if you're after her job. Make no effort at all and you'll be overlooked when it does come to promotion.

★ Hair and make-up do count. Present yourself as a package: hair, make-up and clothes.

★ Every working wardrobe should have a couple of nice shirts. They don't have to be white either – floral, striped or boldly coloured ones look just as fresh.

> ★ Ultimately dress to give your working day a stronger sense of purpose. Think professional rather than (over) powering.

A WORD ON WEEKEND CHIC

What happens to style at the weekend? Women who dress with flair the rest of the week find themselves in tracksuit towelling hell!

Just because these two precious days are supposed to be relaxed doesn't mean you have to be totally off style duty. Unless you have to be suited and booted at work, I think the secret is that whatever you buy for work you can also wear for the weekend. Crossover items would include T-shirts that can be teemed with well-cut trousers, jackets that can be worn with jeans, and crewneck sweaters that are worn with skirts in the week and go with cargo pants at the weekend. Or why not take a dress you would wear to work with a stylish jacket and wear it at the weekend with a fitted denim jacket? The only exception to the rule would be shoes. Flip-flops, for instance, don't really cut it in the boardroom and heels look far too try-hard when worn for a Sunday barbecue.

 TIME TO DITCH *Cheap tights. They look it and can crush a great look.*

 CHANGE IT NOW *Invest in quality tights and your legs will look 100 per cent chicer.*

The basic idea is to whip up a hybrid of style: relaxed but with standout fashion appeal. And if you really can't let go of the tracksuit, at least make it high style. Leisure clothes have recently gone deluxe, so hunt out silk instead of towelling.

 TIME TO DITCH *Designer snobbery.*

 CHANGE IT NOW *Buy it because it looks amazing, not for its label.*

WHEN MAINTENANCE MATTERS

Broken zippers, crumpled clothes and loose buttons dishevel your look before you've even started the day. Maintenance matters and keeping your clothes looking new is one of the smartest things you can do.

★ I cannot overestimate the importance of buying a good steam iron. It will cut your ironing time down by half and leave your clothes looking professionally pressed.

★ Hang and fold your clothes properly to minimise crinkling. Leave at least half an inch of space between hangers to allow your clothes to 'breathe'.

★ Always put away your clothing the minute you take it off. Avoid hanging coats on hooks, as this leaves lumps and indentations and the garment will get out of shape.

★ Read the labels. Note the fabrics and their cleaning requirements. I've lost more than a couple of items to the bin when I've washed instead of dry-cleaned.

★ Always iron your clothes inside out to stop them from becoming shiny.

★ Keep clothes in shape by emptying pockets before hanging them up. Saggy pockets are not a good look.

★ Don't hang knitted garments – it will cause them to stretch out of shape. Fold or roll them instead.

★ Sew a loose button back on immediately. There's nothing more annoying than losing a button and never finding an exact replacement.

★ A laundry basket is vital to good clothes maintenance. Buy one that's big and without the snagging potential (unlined wicker) that can harm delicate items.

★ Handwash extra-delicate items of lingerie.

★ Act quickly on stains. The longer you leave them, the more they will settle. Take your dirty laundry to the cleaner quickly and give a full history of what the stain is and how long it's been on there.

★ Jackets and trousers should rest for a day before being worn again. Rotate all the items in your wardrobe on a daily basis.

★ Dust can prematurely deteriorate your clothes. Brush them regularly with a natural bristle clothes brush.

★ All trousers should be hung using a clamp-style hanger. Folding them over a hanger will only give you a line mid-way down the trouser.

★ Never 'boil' your whites in the washing machine hoping they come out whiter. Years ago clothes were mainly 100 per cent cotton, so could tolerate hot temperatures, but today most garments are cotton mix to help them retain

their shape and will go grey if you boil them.
★ Never overload the washing machine. Detergent residue that cannot be washed away freely causes dinginess.

Feeling fantastic in your underwear

There's nothing worse than comfy washed-out bra syndrome. That's when you just use your underwear to uplift and cover the necessary and keep out the cold!

In my view, underwear denotes the sexiness that a woman conceals beneath her outer garments. And don't be brainwashed into thinking that great-looking underwear is just there to lead a man into temptation. I wear underwear for myself and so should you!

Above all, well-fitting underwear is the foundation that either makes or breaks an outfit. If you wear a bra that is no longer supportive or is too tight and bunching up flesh, even your most expensive clothes won't look flattering.

BRA BUSTING

A bra isn't for life. Although judging by the state some of them are worn in, you would think they were. Generally a bra will last for around three to six months, depending on how often you wear and wash it.

Plus, I'm amazed how many women never remeasure themselves after losing a considerable amount of weight or having babies. Your bra size isn't frozen in time – it changes, whether due to the advancing of years or even something as simple as taking the Pill. That's why it's important you measure yourself or get professionally measured every six months or so.

How to measure yourself: Wearing a bra, put the tape measure snugly around your ribcage, right under your breasts. Read the inches and then add five inches to get your bra size. If the measurement is an odd number, you can either go up for a looser fit or down for a tighter fit.

Now for your cup size: measure around the fullest part of your bust and the difference between the two measurements is your cup size. One inch difference adds up to size A, two inches for B, three inches for C, and so on.

Does your bra fit? Wise up and become a bra connoisseur. Remember the perfect bra with the perfect dress adds up to instant va-va-voom!

Here are guidelines to a great fit:

★ The centre bra panel should rest on your breastbone.
★ The cup should contain the entire breast. Spillage at the top or under the arm does not make for a good fit.
★ The bra should be snug, but not tight. Use the middle set of hooks to fasten it.
★ With a proper fit you should be able to comfortably slide one finger under the band at the front and back of the bra.
★ If the band rides up at the back this is a sign the bra is too large.
★ The straps should not cut into the shoulders. You should

be able to get two fingers under the strap. And adjust them properly so you're not hanging out.

★ The cups should not move your breasts towards the side or the centre. There should be a natural-looking separation of the breasts.

★ The underarm area should lie smooth – the bra should not cut into the flesh.

★ Underwires should not rest on the breast tissue and should fully enclose your bust.

Bosom Buddies (types of bra)

★ *Backless:* Good for halter necks.

★ *Stick-on cups:* Cover your nipples so you can go bra-less.

★ *Convertible:* A bra with removable straps.

★ *Minimiser:* A bra for the woman with a generous bosom who wishes to de-emphasise her bust.

★ *Plunge:* Cut low in front for under a low-cut top.

★ *Push-up:* Pads at the bottom of the cup lift small breasts up.

★ *Soft cup:* This bra has no underwire, so is only for the pert.

★ *Seamless:* No seams across the cup give a smooth, invisible look.

★ *T-shirt bra:* A moulded bra, seamless with double layer cups to prevent nipple show.

KNICKERS!

A very quick word on your smalls: saggy, baggy, grey knickers are a complete turn-off, even if you can't see them. And poorly fitting pants can ruin the line of your clothes.

Whatever type of knickers you choose, whether bikini, brief or high cut, the bottom part should be symmetrical and hug your bum. Otherwise you will be pulling and tugging all day long.

 TIME TO DITCH *Peek-a-boo pants.*

 CHANGE IT NOW *If your trousers are low rise, your pants should be too!*

Necessary accessories

Shoes! Bags! Jewellery! Learn the art of accessorising and you can totally change your look without too much effort.

What I love about accessorising is the way one very small item can totally sex up an otherwise dullish outfit. The cheapest pair of earrings can not only add sparkle to your eyes but seemingly update an outfit you've had for years.

The skill is to think of all these add-ons as part of your wardrobe. Anything overstyled can look cluttered and foolish, so again control comes into play. But invest in the right accessories and wear them with style and you can actually get away with not having to spend a large amount of money on clothes. Yes, really!

For example, a pair of chandelier earrings I hunted out at an antique fayre once are noticeable and exciting enough for people to comment upon them – even strangers. If I have to go to a work function solo, I always wear them, as I guarantee I never end up as Jacqui No Friends for too long. Within a few minutes somebody will always come up to me, primarily to compliment me on my earrings. They make for a great conversation starter.

But just as the right accessories can make your look, so

the wrong ones can break it. Here I've identified key accessories and how to work them to the max.

SHOES

'I don't know who invented high heels, but all women owe him a lot.'

Marilyn Monroe

When buying shoes, we forget pain and start thinking style. I've seen women literally bare their teeth at each other in order to snag the last pair of shoes in their size at a very well-heeled shop. Which just goes to show that if the shoe fits, it's worth fighting for!

It's the Cinderella syndrome. Slip on a pair of decent shoes and you can literally be transported into another fashion world. A high-street skirt can look like couture when worn with fabulous heels.

Shoe Style

I think in every wardrobe these styles of shoes should be included:

★ *Kitten heels:* These make you feel feminine and flirty. More manageable to walk in than a fully blown stiletto, they nevertheless are just as flattering. They go from day to evening effortlessly and even look good with trousers.

★ *Stiletto heels:* They may be hell to wear, but can make the shortest of legs appear longer and an outfit far sexier than you had ever imagined.

★ *Flat pumps:* These look great when worn with narrow and cropped trousers. If wearing them with skirts, make sure the hem drops to the floor or rests above the knee. Any hem in between equals frumpy.

★ *Peep-toed sandals with a heel:* The summer equivalent of kitten heels – but always have a pedicure before wearing them.

★ *Flip-flops:* The humble flip-flop has now elevated itself to a must-have. Just be warned that feet have to be in tip-top condition to pull them off with style.

★ *Boots:* Knee-high boots are a staple and can change an outfit from so-so to seductive. They look great worn with shortish skirts or under trousers or jeans if the heel is high. If you have racehorse legs and are tall, you can even get away with over-the-knee boots. Boots can be an exclamation mark on the most conservative of outfits, so allow yourself a couple of pairs, one of which is extravagant.

A word on comfort: Buy shoes at the end of the day, as your feet will be more swollen then. To test the shoes, as well as walking one or two paces up and down, wriggle your toes and flex your ankles. Avoid synthetic shoes – they'll make your feet sweat.

BAGS

When I say, 'Lose the baggage!', I don't mean a great-looking bag. One bag never fits all looks, so you need a wardrobe of bags and, like shoes, you should have a few styles to call upon.

The mistake many women make when buying bags is they don't 'try them on'. Yes, just like clothes you need to take a couple of minutes twirling in front of a full-length mirror to see how your bag fits.

Bags to Fit

★ If you're five foot nothing, a huge tote bag will do nothing more than make you look smaller.

★ If you're statuesque, a tiny bag can make you look like a giant.

★ The smartest bags flatter your shape. A bag that hits you at your widest part will make you appear dumpy.

★ A woman with a full bosom will find a bag that rests at or below the waist more flattering than a bag that's tucked and nestled against her bust.

★ Women with generous hips should choose a bag that lies under their arm rather than a long-strapped one that nestles on their biggest part.

When shopping for bags, make sure they are big enough for the occasion. An overstuffed evening bag never looks glamorous. When in the shop, empty a bag of all its stuffing so you can get a good idea of how roomy it is inside.

And be frivolous with your bags. Where you can't get away with sequins or bright colours on clothes, you can on bags.

SUNGLASSES

Sunglasses have always symbolised cool. Think of the signature big rounded shades Jackie O wore. But if they're the wrong shape for your face, they'll end up wearing you.

As a general rule, make sure your glasses match your body's proportions and for frames stick to classic black, browns and tortoiseshell. Any other colour shouts 'Clown!'

 TIME TO DITCH *The rock-star coloured lenses.*

 CHANGE IT NOW *Stick to black to save your mystery and dignity.*

If you have striking cheekbones, your glasses shouldn't cover them. If in doubt, opt for oval frames, as they flatter almost any face shape.

SCARVES AND BELTS

Scarves can either look sassy or give the impression you've joined the WI. The skill is in the draping and tying, and that comes with trial and error.

Scarves are very versatile. You can wear them as a neck tie, threaded through belt loops, as a head covering for that racy sports-car look or even beach-sarong style. For all of these styles the scarf needs to be soft and thin. Too starchy and it will go nowhere.

The Scarf Rules

★ Avoid tying knots where they will draw the eye to your largest part.

★ Don't wear a scarf choker style if you have a double chin

★ Match the size of your scarf to the size of your body. A small woman looks ridiculous when swathed in a shawl.

Now for belts. I don't think you should look upon a belt as a figure-enhancing tool. There's nothing worse than seeing someone who's taken a belt and just flung it tightly around their middle in the hope that it will give them a waist. It won't. All it will do is make the hips and bust look bigger.

A great buckle can make an outfit pop, but go for classic dark or matte-finished leather ones rather than coloured leather, as these look the most slimming.

And never be tempted to wear a belt where there are no loops. It rarely ever works unless you're a super-skinny, super-tall model.

Always try a belt on before buying it. You want it to fit into the loops nicely and to make sure it's neither too long nor too short.

JEWELLERY

> 'I adore wearing gems, but not because they're mine. You can't possess radiance, you can only admire it.'
>
> **Elizabeth Taylor**

Wearing jewellery you truly adore is paramount to your style. There are of course your 'precious' jewels – pieces that were bought especially for you by a loved one – but then there's also the jewellery that you buy for yourself. And it needn't cost a fortune.

TIME TO DITCH *Overloading yourself with trinkets so you shine more brightly than the lights on a Christmas tree.*

CHANGE IT NOW *Choose one great piece (real or fake) that can look beautiful when worn on its own. And generally, if you're wearing a 'statement' necklace, ease up on the earrings and vice versa.*

The real beauty of jewellery lies in the way in which you wear it and its ability to make you shine. Long and slender earrings, for instance, can make you feel long and slender too, and a stunning pendant can bring life to the neckline of a plain shirt while enhancing your cleavage.

Signs You're Looking Hot

★ Every guy in your department at the office e-mails you with an urgent 'work' question that needs to be discussed over lunch.

★ The stationmaster tips his hat at you for the first time, even though you've been getting the 8.15 for five years.

★ Your husband says you look great as you leave for work rather than burying his head in the newspaper.

★ You even look good under the loo's harsh, show-the-warts-and-all strip lighting.

Signs You're Not

★ You're asked to cover the phones while everybody else in the office goes out for a lunchtime drink.

★ A person offers you a seat on the tube even though you're not pregnant.

★ Your boss says you look like you need a holiday.

★ You look like a wanted poster (with warts) in the fluorescent lighting in the loo.

GET GORGEOUS: 20 INSTANT STYLE TIPS

1. Wear a bustier whenever you feel the need to turn heads. It instantly gives you an hourglass figure without having to break a sweat at the gym.

2. Until you're confident about your style, avoid seasonal looks. Instead choose quality pieces in simple styles, as you will wear them for longer.

3. Make sure your tights fit correctly. There's nothing worse than the look of wrinkled tights.

4. Look expensive, not cheap. Decide whether you want to show curves or flesh, but never both.

5. If you're worried about clothes clinging in all the wrong places, never buy anything with more than 5 per cent Lycra.

6. The camera never lies. Take a Polaroid in your big-date dress before you wear it. And then decide.

7. A slim V neck will always make your neck look longer.

8. If you always wear trainers, step out in ballet pumps once in a while. They're still flat, but upgrade your style.

9. Get into the habit of wearing dresses. Not many women do, but they're so easy to wear and you can look polished in seconds.

10. Give your look a 24-carat touch by teaming a shimmer shade such as metallic silver with a matt neutral.

11. Never wear pleats if you could do with losing half a stone.

12. A LBD is your safe dress date. Update it by looking for twists in the details such as a gathered bust or a dramatic neckline.

13. If your colour is showy, keep the shape clean.

14. For a bum minimiser, go for an A-line silhouette. This will create the right proportion when worn with a deep-cut top.

15. The straight-leg trouser is an instant leg lengthener. For a lean line, go for a pair with a side fastening and no pockets.

16. Your coat is the first thing anyone sees. Take time in picking the right one for your shape.

17. If you're undecided about something, never be afraid to ask the shop assistant to put it on hold. You can then think about it for a day and go back.

18. Think about hiring a personal shopper. They're a free service with large department stores and can give you the confidence you need to makeover your look.

19. Choose exquisite fabrics to make yourself look special. Velvets, silk, cashmere and lace all feel seductive when worn against the skin.

20. Don't shy away from all-over prints. They can look extremely modern and actually keep the eye moving away from areas you'd rather they didn't focus on.

Resources

UK HOT SPOTS

Hair Salons
Richard Ward
162b Sloane Street
London SW1
Tel: +44 (0)20 7245 6151

Colourist
Jo Hansford
19 Mount Street
London W1Y 5RA
Tel: +44 (0)20 7495 7774

Teeth Whitening
Capital Dental
Tel: +44 (0)800 587 7962

BriteSmile
Tel: +44 (0)800 076 8768

Facialist
Leonard Drake Skin Care
Centres
8 Lancer Square
Kensington Church Street
London W8 4EH
Tel: +44 (0)20 7937 7060
and
The Cloisters Mall
Kingston upon Thames
Surrey KT1
Tel: +44 (0)20 8541 0999

Fitness
David Lloyd Leisure
family-friendly fitness
centres that have 57 clubs
across the UK and Ireland.
Tel: +44 (0)870 888 3015
www.davidlloydleisure.co.uk

Esporta Fitness Clubs
All clubs have a well-
equipped fitness arena and
swimming pools.
Tel: +44 (0)870 739 0039
www.esporta.com

Body Control Pilates
Tel: +44 (0)20 7379 3734
www.bodycontrol.co.uk

Nutrition
The Institute of Optimum
Nutrition
Tel: +44 (0)20 8874 9427
for a nutritionist in your
area.

AUSTRALIAN HOT SPOTS
Spas
Jurlique Wellness
Sanctuary Day Spa
Como Centre
Chapel Street
Toorak Road
South Yarrow
Melbourne
Tel +61 (0)3 9827 0755

Spa Chakra
6 Cowper Wharf Road
Woolloomooloo
New South Wales
www.chakra.net.spa

Hair Salon
Valonz Haircutters
10 William Street
Paddington
Sydney
Tel: +61 (0)293 602 444

Beauty Junkie Store
Miss Frou Frou
20–22 Elizabeth Street
Paddington
Sydney
Tel: + 61 (0)293 602 869

Hair Removal
The Australian Laser Clinic
www.laserclinic.com.au

NEW ZEALAND HOT SPOTS
Day Spa
L'unova
48 Broadway
Newmarket
Auckland
Tel: +64 (0)9 520 6731

Hairdresser

Glint
159 Hurstmere Road
Takapuna
North Shore
Auckland
Tel: +64 (0)9 489 9058

Best Store for Beauty Junkies

Glamourpuss
290a Broadway
Newmarket
Auckland
Tel: +64 (0)9 524 4741

SOUTH AFRICAN HOT SPOTS

Health & Beauty Clinic

Aromabar
23 Derry Street
Vredehoek
Cape Town
Tel: +27 (0)21 461 66 10

Spa

S.K.I.N Wellness Spa
Dock Road
V&A Waterfront
Cape Town
Tel: +27 (0)21 425 3 551
www.skinonline.co.za

Hair Salon

Isjon Intercoiffure
Tel: + 27 (0)11 805 4655

Cosmetic Surgeon

Dr Des Fernandes
822 Fountain Medical Centre
Heerengracht Centre
Cape Town
Tel: + 27 (0)21 425 2310

Index